Ketogenic Diet: What It Is And How It Works:

The Diet That Uses Fat As An Energy Source

Author Name
Alexia Keto

Table of Contents

12. Conclusion

Introduction

Congratulations on purchasing *Ketogenic Diet: What It Is And How It Works* and thank you for doing so.

There are plenty of books on this subject on the market, thanks again for choosing this one! Every effort was made to ensure it is full of as much useful information as possible, please enjoy!

Ketogenic diets are on everyone's lips, but usually, the implementation fails simply because a sound knowledge of ketogenic nutrition is missing. On the Internet, many keto recipes are published today, which would fall under the category of low carb maximum. Ketogenic diets and low carb diets are of course closely related, with a keto diet called 'No Carb' rather appropriate. Carbohydrates, carbs, are largely dispensed within this diet. In the first chapter, we would like to focus intensely on what distinguishes a ketogenic diet and what causes it.

Chapter 1 - The Ketogenic Diet - What Is Behind It?

The principle is actually very simple. Once the body is given very few carbohydrates, they can no longer be used to generate energy, and the body is looking for an alternative solution on its own. Due to the alleged deficiency, so-called ketogens are produced from fats in the liver and used as an energy source. This body-own procedure is called Ketose and is the A and O - with a ketogene nutrition. The big goal is to bring the body in the so-called Ketose. While the carbohydrates are drastically reduced, the consumption of fat is relatively high. Generally, the rule of thumb is that 5% of the diet should consist of carbohydrates, 35% protein, and 60% fat. In order to avoid cravings, it is particularly important during a ketogenic diet that the recipes are varied. Only if the diet is colorful and multifaceted even during a diet, the loss of weight will be successful in the long term. Of course, according to the ketogenic method, you could only feed for days on fried meat and eggs. This is just as effective, but this diet will sooner or later hang over your throat and you give up. Also, one-sided nutrition is not proven to be healthy. With our recipes, your body gets all the vitamins, minerals and trace elements, as well as fiber, which it needs. So you stay healthy and vital during the diet.

What Foods Are On The Prohibited "Black List"?

All foods that contain many carbohydrates are of course banned. But do not worry, in our recipes you will find great alternatives. Noodles, rice, and legumes are, however, consistently removed from the diet. Also, potatoes, sweet potatoes, and carbohydrate-rich root vegetables are omitted. Of course, soft drinks like Coke and Pepsi are also deleted. Many people think that fruit juices are very healthy, but they also contain too much sugar and are, therefore, a no-go. Diet sugar-free sweetened drinks are allowed. Even fruit itself is on the blacklist. Only berries in small quantities are allowed- and those too, not every day.

During the ketogenic diet should be consistently dispensed with alcohol. Alcohol not only has a lot of calories and carbohydrates but after consuming alcohol, the appetite for sweet, fat and unhealthy foods increases.

Too much salt and finished products, including spice mixtures, should be avoided. Especially in spice mixtures, people often hide a lot of sugar. You should get used to reading the declarations of the packaging carefully. For example, yogurts are often referred to as light or diet. These are usually reduced only by fat and still contain a lot of sugar. So grab the products that have a high-fat content, but are without added sugar.

Which Foods Are Allowed?

Meat, fish and seafood, eggs and dairy products are high on the list during a ketogenic diet. Nuts, seeds, herbs and especially high-quality oils are also allowed. With vegetables, you should resort to variants with few carbohydrates. These include avocados, tomatoes, onions and, above all, all green vegetables now dominate your diet.

To sweeten, you can use ordinary sweetener from the trade, but you can also take to stevia, xylitol or birch sugar. Honey is also not allowed during the ketogenic diet and maple syrup is also deleted.

What Is So Special About The Ketogenic Diet?

The big advantage of this diet is that the body decreases pretty quickly and the pounds nearly fall during sleep. A big plus in comparison to many other weight loss programs is that no calories or points need to be counted here. Also, it is not necessary to measure all food exactly with the scale. The only thing that counts is that the foods contain as few carbohydrates as possible. If this is followed, this diet is really effective.

The blood sugar level is kept constant low and after a few days, the appetite for sweets disappears. Sugar and carbohydrates are similar to those of alcohol or nicotine, but only very few people are aware of it. If this is done consistently, the cravings fade away after just a few days. Since you can really eat enough with this diet, your thoughts are not always about the next meal. This is a big plus to be able to really endure a diet.

Of course, a diet should always be started after consultation with the doctor. However, the ketogenic diet has also been very successful in patients with diabetes in the past, and even heart patients, epileptics and even Alzheimer's patients have been able to successfully and healthily lose weight with this diet. Consuming low sugar can also improve skin conditions and even acne. Therefore, the keto diet is especially recommended for adolescents in puberty.
Are There Any Disadvantages To The Ketogenic Diet?

In addition to a strong craving for sugar in the first few days which disappears quite quickly, it can initially cause an increased headache. But this pain is good to counteract. It is important that enough water is being drunk. Water is not only important to flush out the toxins. Those who drink enough automatically reduce the feeling of hunger. If you have problems with gout and uric acid, you should definitely clarify the diet plan with the attending physician in advance.

But now, we do not want to torture you anymore and start with our recipes. This little guide is divided into categories for breakfast, lunch, and dinner, snacks, drinks, and desserts. Afterwards, you will also find a plan for a 14-day program. There we prepared two meals each, which you can combine as you wish with a breakfast or a snack. Always make sure that your total carbohydrate turnover is no more than 20 grams to a maximum of 30 grams.

Burning Fat

A hot tip for maximum fat burning during sleep is the protein booster. The recipe can be found in our chapter snacks. This you can taste just before going to bed. It boosts your metabolism and your pounds melt away overnight.

So that you do not get seduced in between, you should optimize your fridge and the pantry in advance and all " sins " leave your field of vision. This is a little trick with a big impact because everything that does not exist can not tempt you either.

For many years now, I have been studying everything that is in any way connected with our health. I hope this story helps you avoid those painful stupid mistakes that I made on my long journey to the goal because it is much better and easier to learn from the mistakes of others than from my own.

My passion for fitness began in 1968. Dr. Ken Cooper's book, Aerobics, inspired me to take care of my health, and ten years later - to go to medical school. Unfortunately, like many fans of healthy eating in the late 1960s and early 1970s, I was on a low-fat, high-carb diet that has not lost its popularity for decades. In fact, this type of diet is the exact opposite of the one that can protect us from chronic diseases, defeat cancer and optimize health.

During years of studying at a medical school and family practice in residency, I was hammered into the traditional medical model of drug treatment, which is mainly aimed at eliminating the symptoms of the disease. In fact, for all these years of study, I have never once turned to the root cause of chronic disorders. It was only working with symptoms using pharmaceuticals and medical procedures.

In 1995, in my mind, came a real revolution. I met Dr. Ron Rosdale among other doctors at a meeting at Great Lake Medical Academy. Then I still did not understand how lucky I was, because I was one of the first to draw inspiration from the scientific research of Dr. Rosdale in the field of clinical metabolic biochemistry.

For more than three hours, Dr. Rosdale gave a lecture on the need to control high levels of insulin in the blood in order to prevent the emergence of many chronic degenerative diseases that have become a real epidemic in recent years: diabetes, obesity, cardiovascular disease, oncology, and arthritis, and neurodegenerative disorders.

You have probably ever found truth in your life and experienced a sense of insight. In this case, I understood that what I heard and what most beneficially affected my health, affects hundreds of millions of people and they are so in need of help.

Over the next ten years, I used not only the principles that Dr. Rosdale taught me but also the knowledge I received in all kinds of nutrition courses for graduate students. I must say that in a medical school such a subject as nutrition did not teach me. Thus, my idea of food as a medicine gradually developed. (And today in most medical schools students are not even taught the basics of nutrition.

It's a big reward for me to lend a helping hand to those who could not be cured by leading experts in the best institutes of the country. Do not think that I consider myself smarter than these doctors. In no case, that exists.

I differ from them only in that I always persistently and purposefully seek answers to questions regarding our health with you. The secret is simple. I stopped satisfying the interests of pharmacists and concentrated on the body's ability to heal itself. Thus, I managed the main thing - not to alleviate the symptoms of the disease, but to eliminate the causes of its occurrence. At that time, I already realized the need to limit refined carbohydrates and processed foods and find a substitute for them, but I still had no idea about the importance of consuming high-quality fats and activating the body's natural ability to burn them as the main source of energy. I did not even suspect what a long way I still had to go.

We lose in the war on cancer because for many years we fought the wrong enemy. Twenty years after I learned about the important role of insulin, I happened to read Travis Kristofferson's book "Walking the Truth: How the Metabolic Cancer Theory Turns Over the Most Common Paradigms in Medicine". I felt the same sense of insight that I had once experienced in Dr. Rosdale's lecture. Here it is, saving the lives of millions of people! Kristofferson's theory (in my head it was superimposed on what Dr. Rosdale taught me in 1995) is that oncology and most chronic diseases result from metabolic disturbances in mitochondria. Usually this is due to the resistance (immunity) of insulin and leptin receptors when consuming a high proportion of pure carbohydrates and the activation of metabolic signaling pathways due to excess protein. I will tell you about the details a bit later, now you just need to understand what is the cause of many problems.

According to the accepted scientific dogma, cancer is a genetic disease that occurs as a result of a chromosomal disorder in the nuclei of a cell. Watson's discovery of the DNA structure was a cry in the middle of the twentieth century and subsequent studies in the twenty-first century contributed to the rethinking of obsolete views.

All this is the exact opposite of traditional views that have existed for more than a century. Unfortunately, the cancer war launched by President Nixon with the signing of the National Cancer Act in 1971 was a complete failure. In 2016, they waited for the innovations of President Obama. Despite multi-billion dollar investments, now in the United States of America alone, more than 1,600 people die from cancer per day. If we look at world statistics, this figure rises to terrifying - 21,000 people a day. Every day, 21,000 people worldwide die of cancer. But these statistics can be changed. Recent discoveries confirm: oncology is not DNA damage, it is a metabolic disorder.

In most cases, the disease can be prevented. The colossal scale of the epidemic suggests that one day, you or someone close to you can get cancer. It is shocking, but the data for the period 2011-2013 show that 40% of us will sooner or later hear a terrible diagnosis. I am here to say: we are losing the war with oncology because scientists are following the wrong paradigm. The cause of cancer in most adults is not DNA damage, but a metabolic disorder.

Chapter 2 - Omnipotent Mitochondria

Mitochondria are tiny "plants" inside cells that use metabolic processes to process the food you eat and the air you absorb into energy. They are the root cause of disturbances in the biological system, increasing the risk of cancer and chronic diseases. When most mitochondria begin to malfunction, the body simply cannot stay healthy. This is a big shift in our understanding of oncology and all chronic diseases. If the cause is metabolic dysfunction, then it must be eliminated. How? After reading the book, you will learn how to choose nutrients and use other methods that will allow you to "enable" the body's ability to defend itself and recover from the disease.

Speaking accessible, the theory proposed in my book is based on the fact that everyday food preferences have a great influence on the state of mitochondria. If you eat foods that are beneficial for mitochondria, the genetic material contained in them will not be affected, the chain reaction will not start, and you will maintain your health.

Another reason I started writing this book was the large number of friends and colleagues who died of cancer, including Jerry Burnetti. Without exaggeration: Jerry was a genius. He was one of the world's leading experts in regenerative farming. I had a happy opportunity several years ago to interview him for a number of websites.

The film "Guilty Stars", a heartbreaking romantic drama about two teenagers with cancer who meet and fall in love despite the fact that they are destined to die soon, inspired me and became one of my favorites. If you have not watched it or read the book on which it was shot, be sure to do it.

I believe, like everyone with whom I spoke, preparing this book for publication: tragic scenarios like Jerry's early death and what we see in the film can be avoided. After all, more than 90% of cases of cancer can be prevented or cured. I just had to take measures to save so much from a terrible diagnosis.

After watching the film and reading Travis's book, I went to the National Library of Medicine for the latest research, which later led me to hundreds of articles on the important role of mitochondria and the various factors to improve their functioning. I was able to understand this topic by communicating with many reputable experts in this field.

I would especially like to highlight Miriam Kalamian, Ed.M., MS, C.NS, nutrition consultant, educator, author of books on the use of ketogenic therapy in cancer patients. Miriam often helps out with the advice of Dr. Thomas Seyfried, one of the first to use mitochondrial metabolic therapy to treat cancer. She helped and helps hundreds of patients switch to my diet, and also provided useful information that you should familiarize yourself with. This book is like a big puzzle made of pieces of information, and Miriam helped me assemble this puzzle.

A Nutrition Program That Helps Establish Metabolism

The purpose of the book is to provide a clear, simple, and rational explanation, backed up by scientific evidence, to help you understand how the body functions at the biological and molecular levels. I will tell you what to eat, what practical strategies to follow and how to track your own successes on the path to healing mitochondria. I called this program mitochondrial metabolic therapy or MMT for short.

In short, MMT is a nutritional system that will rebuild metabolism and replace the main fuel for your body from glucose to fats. In this way, mitochondrial function is optimized and their DNA will become more protected from damage that contributes to the emergence of diseases.

Mitochondrial metabolic therapy is not just a diet, it is important WHAT you eat and WHEN, since regular fasting helps improve mitochondrial function and it is easier to rebuild the body to burn fat instead of glucose (do not be afraid, we will only starve at night). The basis of MMT is a high-fat, low-carb, moderately protein-rich diet, which is based on the consumption of high-quality products. This is not a typical American diet, famous for a large share of refined grains, sugars, and low-quality fats. You will see for yourself that the food at the heart of MMT is very tasty, even exquisite. It saturates the body and fills it with energy. And when you finally go to MMT, then get rid of hunger, craving for food and deprivation – faithful companions to most power modes and falsehoods.

MMT is designed for those who suffer from one or more serious diseases, including oncology, type 2 diabetes, neurodegenerative diseases (Alzheimer's disease) and other forms of dementia, as well as obesity. Therapy is also suitable for those people who want to optimize their health and slow down the aging process. MMT has no strict framework. The choice is always wonderful. Perhaps at the moment you do not consider yourself to be classified either as chronically ill or as supporters of a healthy lifestyle. But when you have a desire to take care of your health, you will already have a powerful weapon in your hands against many problems. It costs a lot.

This is just an emerging science but you can take advantage of its fruits even now. You must understand that mitochondrial and metabolic health is a nascent discipline, and at the moment there are only a few researchers and even fewer practitioners who apply these developments. But I am firmly convinced that one day, metabolic therapy will become an accepted standard of treatment not only for oncology but also for most chronic diseases.

Thank God you and your family do not need to wait ten or twenty years for this event. You can improve your health right now, prevent unnecessary pain and suffering, and reduce the risk of developing chronic diseases, including oncology, using the current knowledge about mitochondrial dysfunctions. I am fully aware that most of the information in this book is not generally accepted and is likely to be harshly criticized. But I and everyone else who advocates a comprehensive view of human health and treatment is already accustomed to such a reaction. After all, we offer a more rational and safe way to not get sick.

There are many examples in history when the routine use of pharmaceuticals and other medical interventions are considered "treatment standards" until someone proves their failure and danger to health.

I first encountered this in the early 1980s when I was in medical school. Instead of using drugs to treat ulcers, I advised taking measures to improve intestinal microflora. A new idea came across a general misunderstanding and condemnation from my teachers. Years later, this method became the standard of treatment. I made sure that I was absolutely right. Dr. Barry Marshall was that talented family doctor who directed me on the right path, and 25 years later, in 2005, he received the Nobel Prize in medicine.

Then I was one of the first who openly declared the dangers of the anti-inflammatory drug Vioxx. The year before the drug was approved for use in the United States, I informed my site readers that it can cause cardiovascular disease and even a heart attack. Four years after the appearance of Vioxx on pharmacy shelves, the pharmaceutical company Merch arbitrarily withdrew the drug before it could kill 60,000 people.

I believe that the time has come to challenge accepted views on the causes of cancer and methods of treatment. We must become more open and revise modern theories, because science never stands still, as, in fact, our understanding of biology.

At first, I did not want to write a book about mitochondrial dysfunction and oncology, because the information in this area is becoming obsolete at a rapid pace. I thought it was much better and more useful to publish real-time information on the Internet on my website, which I launched in 1997 and conducted in my free time. Gradually, this site has become one of the most popular in the world: more than 15 million visitors and 40 million views per month. But my friends and colleagues convinced me ten years ago that books have a special mission: to write them, the author must fit his thoughts into a comprehensive print resource, where all the material is presented in a format that is easy to understand.

I am convinced that the information presented in this book will definitely need to be reviewed in the near future. But in order for the need to completely rewrite it, many years must pass. That is why I urge you to keep up with the latest science news. It is my great happiness to see how, thanks to this information, people get hope and begin to take care of their health without the use of potentially dangerous and toxic pharmaceuticals. I hope that my book will help many, many more.

The Truth About Mitochondria, Free Radicals, and Dietary Fats

If you are reading this book, I dare to suggest that you are aware of the connection between what you eat and how you feel; you yourself or someone you love has faced the problem of poor-quality medical care at least once.

I'm almost sure that you have finally ceased to understand what food is considered useful. Indeed, it is very difficult not to get confused when the food and pharmaceutical industries, having learned to speak beautifully, bypass laws all the time. They easily distort the truth in pursuit of profit. They systematically and deliberately introduce you to misconceptions regarding the harm and health benefits of certain products. I spend most of my free time studying scientific papers and communicating with leading experts in various fields. Having a family doctor diploma and many years of experience working with patients — more than 25,000 people — I constantly try to rethink and refine my own idea of a healthy diet.

In this chapter, I will try to explain the meaning of several key terms, so that, moving on to the second part of the book, you can understand why the nutritional system that I offer is really able to restore health and prevent many diseases. First of all, it should be understood what mitochondria are, why fats of one type are your allies, and fats of another type are enemies, what stages of cleavage they go through and, finally, what recommendations in the field of dietetics are worth trusting and which ones are not. I hope that by the end of the chapter you will realize why it is so important to take care of mitochondria and how the traditional American diet can harm these tiny "bricks" of the body.

It is possible that you heard about mitochondria in biology classes in high school or read on the Internet about mitochondrial disease, and yet you still do not fully understand what it is and what their function is. Mitochondria are extremely important for maintaining health, so if you want to protect yourself or recover from illnesses, you just need to learn as much about them as possible.

Mitochondria are tiny organelles (similar to microorganisms), they are present in almost all cells. One of their most important functions is the production of energy by combining the nutrients from glucose and the fats you consume with the oxygen you breathe. Mitochondria are the "batteries" of your cells. They help generate energy by combining nutrients with oxygen. Mitochondria account for 10% of the total body weight, and their number in adult cells is approximately 10 million. If it's hard for you to appreciate such an impressive figure, then imagine that more than 1 billion mitochondria can fit on the end of a pin.

Some cells contain more mitochondria than others. The female reproductive cell, called the oocyte, includes hundreds of thousands of mitochondria, while in the mature forms of red blood cells and skin cells they are practically absent. Most cells, including liver cells, contain between 80 and 2,000 mitochondria. The higher the metabolic activity of cells - and such cells are found in the heart, brain, liver, kidneys, and muscles - the more mitochondria they have. Now you can well imagine what an extensive favorable spectrum of action on the whole body is exerted by healthy, properly functioning mitochondria.

Mitochondria constantly produce energy molecules called adenosine triphosphates (ATP). You, as I once did, are probably interested in knowing their exact number. You will be very surprised to learn that your mitochondria produce 110 pounds of ATP per day.

Every second, your body's mitochondria produce 10,000 times more energy than the sun! So you can well appreciate the key role of healthy mitochondria in proper metabolism. Eliminating mitochondrial dysfunction is the easiest and most promising way to restore health and prevent a number of serious diseases, mainly cancer.

Chapter 3 - Free Radicals

Every cell in your body needs a constant influx of energy. The largest amount of energy is produced by mitochondria in a process that combines the two main biological functions of the body necessary to maintain life: respiration and food. This process is scientifically called oxidative phosphorylation; as a result, energy is generated in the form of ATP. (This process is not the main energy production mechanism for cancer cells, where glucose metabolism occurs outside the mitochondria and energy is less actively generated as a result of glycolysis.)

ATP, the "unit of energy", activates absolutely all the biological functions of the body - from the brain to the heartbeat. A heart cell contains more than 5,000 mitochondria. This is the most energetically powerful tissue of our body!

The process of oxidative phosphorylation in mitochondria involves a series of chemical reactions that are difficult to understand even for biochemistry students. They are called the Krebs cycle and the electron transport chain. Together, these two reactions involve electrons that are released from consumed food and protons. The result is continuous energy production. At the end of the chain, electrons react with oxygen and form water.

Part of the electrons will flow out of the electron transport chain, forming reactive oxygen species (ROS). ROS are weak, fragile molecules containing oxygen atoms that have one or more unpaired electrons. These highly reactive atoms form free radicals that can cause destructive processes. Many of you are probably already familiar with this term - "free radicals". Maybe you even believe that they carry a great danger, and try to neutralize them with antioxidants. (I will explain to you why this is not always correct.)

What Is The Harm Of Free Radicals?

Free radicals react with other molecules, resulting in oxidation, the purpose of which is to neutralize an unstable electric charge. Oxidation is essentially "biological corrosion." It creates the effect of a snowball, that is, molecules steal electrons from each other, becoming new free radicals during the bloody biological struggle. The rapidly growing amount of free radicals leads to the destruction of both the cell itself and the mitochondrial membranes. This process is called lipid peroxidation. It causes the fragility of membranes and their decay.

Studies have revealed that DNA is attacked by free radicals from about 10,000 to 100,000 times a day, that is, one negative effect per second. Free radicals can also harm your DNA, disrupting replication processes, interfering with their functioning mechanisms and changing their structure. All these factors cause tissue degradation, as a result of which the risk of getting sick is growing inexorably. In fact, free radicals cause more than 60 different diseases, including the following:

- Alzheimer's disease;
- Atherosclerosis and heart disease;
- oncology;
- cataract;
- Parkinson's disease.

As you have already understood, free radicals have a huge impact on your health. And the most surprising is that approximately 90% (or more) of reactive oxygen species (ROS) are formed in mitochondria. However, it should be remembered that free radicals are not only enemies of our health, but also friends.

Useful Functions Of Free Radicals

They regulate a number of vital cellular functions, such as the production of melanin and nitric oxide, the optimization of metabolic signaling pathways, which are responsible for hunger, fat deposition, and aging. They serve as natural biological signals, arising in response to external stimuli, for example toxins and chemicals in tobacco smoke or air.

They are responsible for the anticancer effect of chemotherapy drugs aimed at stimulating the body's prooxidant system. They contribute to a positive effect on the body of physical activity, as a result of which your body produces more free radicals. The reason for this is the active generation of energy by mitochondria.

Therefore, one should not try to avoid reactive oxygen species (RFC). It is not RFK that is harmful, but their excess in your body. You can resort to MMT to optimize the increase or decrease in RFC in cells. Think of it as a lifesaver. Not too much, not too little RFK, only the right amount produced by healthy mitochondria. Thus, if you diligently suppress free radicals, then most likely, unwillingly, you will earn serious complications.

Reducing the number of free radicals by consuming antioxidant supplements is harmful! This can lead to serious health problems, including the development of oncology. One example of the undesirable effects of excessive consumption of antioxidants is the neutralization of such important ROS or cancer cell mitochondria. Lining up, free radicals lead to self-destruction of cancer cells as a result of apoptosis (programmed cell death process).

If you have been diagnosed with cancer, contact your healthcare provider to limit the number of antioxidants prescribed to you, including vitamins C, E, selenium, and especially N-acetylcysteine. This will greatly contribute to the death of cancer cells. Although it is worth considering that a high dose of vitamin C intravenously or oral liposomal vitamin C is used by many oncologists to treat cancer, and after all, vitamin C tends to turn into hydrogen peroxide, which kills cancer cells.

No additives. We limit the proportion of free radicals to help with the diet. How to maintain the necessary balance of AFC? Fortunately, the answer is very simple. Instead of suppressing excess free radicals with antioxidants, it is better to make sure that your body produces less of them.
That is why what you eat is so important. The main advantage of a diet high in high-quality fats, a low proportion of digestible carbohydrates (carbohydrates minus fiber) and a moderate amount of protein is the optimization of the ability of mitochondria to produce fuel called ketones. They, coupled with low blood glucose, produce much less ROS and secondary free radicals than when you eat mostly carbohydrates.

Carbohydrates are the main reason for the production of a large number of free radicals in your body. In other words, carbohydrates compared to fats can be regarded as dirty fuel. When you eat a low-fat, high-carb diet and burn fats and ketones instead of glucose to generate energy, your mitochondria is 30–40% less oxidized than with sugar, which is typical for our typical diet. Thus, if you are "fat-adapting", that is, you choose fats as the main fuel of the body, your cell membranes, mitochondrial DNA and protein will remain strong, healthy, and stable.

In order to teach the body to burn ketones as the main fuel, you must increase the intake of healthy fats and reduce the proportion of carbohydrates, thereby lowering the level of glucose in the blood. This is the main point of mitochondrial metabolic therapy (MMT).

The only difficulty is the process of replacing carbohydrates with fats, which should be carried out with caution. The fats you choose should be of high quality and best of all - organic. And no industrially processed vegetable oils enriched with omega-6.

You probably already noticed that a high-fat diet is not at all the accepted nutritional schemes and guidelines for a healthy lifestyle but they have not lost their popularity over the past half-century. Thank God, albeit slowly, but the situation is changing. And yet, in order to boldly and competently break the accepted commandments of dietetics, we should look back and understand the reasons for their occurrence.

Well, let's go back to the very beginning of the 20th century to understand how the American revolution in nutrition has affected the whole world.

America In The Early 1900s

At the end of the 19th century, most Americans were either farmers or members of rural communities who ate farm products. There were only a few industrial product companies: in 1898 Kellog's began to produce corn flakes, Heinz, Libby's and Campbell's had long been selling canned goods, and in 1899, Wesson Oil deodorized cottonseed oil appeared on the markets. Nevertheless, most of the products on our tables were local, whole and not subjected to technological processing. It is worth considering that with all this they were still completely natural because synthetic fertilizers and pesticides simply did not exist.

Cottonseed oil before appearing in American cuisines in a bottle labeled Wesson, was considered a waste of the cotton industry and was mainly used in the manufacture of soap and fuel for lamps. With the spread of electricity at the beginning of the 20th century, manufacturers faced the problem of an excess of cotton oil and tried to find use for it.

Unprocessed cottonseed oil has a cloudy structure and a reddish tint due to the content of gossypol, a natural phytochemical that is toxic to animals. Manufacturers had to develop special flavors to make it edible. At one time, an article was published in the Popular Science magazine in the "Opening of the Century" column that very accurately described the path that cottonseed oil took before getting to our table: "Waste - in 1860, fertilizer - in 1870, livestock feed - in 1880, and, finally, a useful food supplement and not only in 1889".

Processing cottonseed oil has not yet made it suitable for consumption. The difficulty was that, like most vegetable oils, it is a polyunsaturated fatty acid (PUFA), and this indicates the presence of multiple (particle "poly-") double bonds of atoms in its molecular structure (while the atoms are "unsaturated") . These double bonds are susceptible to free radical attacks, which gradually damage the molecule. When you consume too much PUFA, their proportion in cell membranes increases significantly. The unstable structure of these fats causes fragility of cells and their predisposition to oxidation, which, in turn, is the cause of a number of diseases, including chronic inflammation and atherosclerosis.

Instability is the main cause of rancidity in vegetable oils. This circumstance repelled many food producers, because with the advent of railways and cold rooms, products began to be transported over long distances and lay on shelves for weeks. Therefore, hydrogenated fats have become a salvation: they eliminated weak double bonds and increased the shelf life of vegetable oils.

In 1910, P&G patented Crisco hydrogenated cottonseed oil, the first trans-fat in the history, launching the process of transition from animal fats to processed fats. In 1907, the German chemist Edwin Kaiser contacted the Procter & Gamble soap company (Cincinnati), claiming that he was able to develop a method for producing liquid fats with a long shelf life. The company bought his rights from him and began to experiment, wanting to make soap cheaper and more attractive in appearance.

With the advent of hydrogenated cottonseed oil, P&G experts noticed that with its white glowing color it resembles lard - the most popular cooking oil of those years. Then why is it still not in our kitchens?

When Procter & Gamble introduced Crisco to the general public in 1911, they called their new product "ideal fat," notable for its "environmental friendliness" and "plant origin". As a result, Crisco sales jumped from 2.6 million pounds to 60 million in four years. In 1909, an ordinary American consumed no more than 9 pounds of industrial processed fats, including margarine and vegetable oil, and by 1950 this figure had risen to 20 pounds per year, where 15 were hydrogenated oils and 5 were vegetable. All varieties of oils, including soybean and corn, were hydrogenated and went on sale in the form of Crisco, margarine and all kinds of packaged, frozen and fried foods.

We began to consume omega-6-rich vegetable oils more than ever in the history of mankind. The three subsequent technical discoveries also had a significant impact on what we eat: synthetic fertilizers, food additives and pesticides (mainly Roundup).

Synthetic fertilizers have been developed to help farmers harvest large crops from a small number of crop varieties. Synthetic fertilizers killed microbes, disrupting the mineralization of the soil, as a result, lands began to appear that were unable to produce crops with high nutritional value.

It has also become possible for farmers to concentrate on growing one or two crops, such as corn and soy, instead of using the traditional method of alternating a large number of different crops in order to prevent soil depletion. Thus, the growing supply of vegetable oils created a demand for them.

Nutritional supplements quickly burst into our lives in the first half of the 20th century. By 1985, about 800 food additives were used. This was done absolutely uncontrollably and without any preliminary studies of their safety. Consumer complaints about the side effects of drugs and food have led Congress to amend the law on food additives. Thus, manufacturers were required to confirm the safety of any food additives before a product hit the store shelves.

But the loophole still remained: additives that received "safe" GRAS status or were widely used before 1958 could be freely used in production without approval or at least from the Food and Drug Administration (FDA). Today out of 10,000 chemicals used in food production, at least 1000 have never been reviewed by the FDA.

Even those additives that are not on the GR AS list often remain unexplored due to the fact that the FDA allows companies to conduct their own research. One glaring example of this negligence in relation to food additives is a priori recognition of safe trans fats. Today, we all know that trans fats contribute to inflammation and increase the risk of heart disease, insulin resistance, obesity, and Alzheimer's disease. The farther, the worse.

Glyphosate - the main active ingredient in the toxic Roundup herbicide - is a serious threat to the health of your mitochondria. Since many vegetable oils, as well as a number of processed foods, are made from genetically modified corn, soy, and canola, they are highly likely to become infected with this chemical. Terribly, about 10 million tons of glyphosate were dumped into the soil from 1974 to 2016.
These are world statistics.
Glyphosate harms your mitochondria in two ways.
In the first case, manganese is a mineral, which in small amounts helps the body maintain bone health and neutralize free radicals. Glyphosate binds manganese and many other important minerals in plants treated with Roundup. Thus, when you eat these plants, you get no benefit. Glyphosate can also bind and remove these minerals from the body. The circumstance is rather unpleasant, because your mitochondria require manganese to turn superoxide, a potentially dangerous by-product of oxygen metabolism, into water. This is an extremely important process that protects mitochondria from oxidation. Without manganese, it is seriously disturbed.

Glyphosate disrupts the process of ATP production, affecting mitochondrial membranes. When glyphosate adheres to so-called inert solvents as part of Roundup, its toxicity increases 2000 times. The membrane structure becomes porous, and glyphosate easily penetrates the very heart of mitochondria.

Chapter 4 – Saturated Fats
Saturated Fats Become Our Enemies

An interesting fact: despite the manufacturers' promises that refined vegetable oil is good for health, the world community in the first half of the 20th century faced a wave of cardiovascular diseases. Although oils have become a new food supplement, it never occurred to anyone to blame them for the problems that arose. A familiar and common useful substance has come under suspicion in a spontaneous and biased study of one person.

The "Great" Study Of Dr. Kies

Fear of fat arose in 1951, when physiology professor Ansel Kies went to Europe to look for the cause of heart disease. Kies heard that in Naples, (Italy), according to statistics, the least people suffering from cardiovascular diseases, so he wanted to observe the eating habits of Neapolitans.

Do not forget that Europe suffered greatly during the Second World War. Its entire infrastructure was destroyed, and for many years after the accession of the world, the threat of hunger remained high. These conditions were especially felt in Greece and Italy, where, according to statistics from 1951, there was less food per capita than in other European countries. Kies took these unusual temporary circumstances as an old tradition and called the "Mediterranean diet."

In Naples, Kies noted that the locals mostly eat pasta and plain pizza for lunch, vegetables sprinkled with olive oil, cheese, fruit for dessert, lots of wine and very little meat. "Only a small class of wealthy people ... ate meat every day, and not once a week or once every two weeks, " he wrote.

Kies's wife, a medical technologist, conducted an unofficial study of Neapolitan blood serum cholesterol and found that it was extremely low for everyone except for Rotary Club members — wealthy people who could afford to buy meat. This completely "unscientific" scientific study led Kies to the idea that the lack of meat in the diet helps to avoid heart attacks. But the predominance of cheese in the diet (also a source of saturated fats) escaped his attention, but later he himself admits that he often overlooks important details.

After Italy, Keyes continued to search for evidence that consuming saturated fats increases the risk of heart disease. He collected data from six countries with a high incidence of heart disease and diets, traditionally consisting of a large amount of saturated fat. The evidence seemed convincing, even logical. For example, mortality among men in America, where traditionally consume a lot of saturated fats, was higher than the mortality of men in Japan, where the proportion of saturated fats in the diet is much lower.

But there was some unevenness. Kies did not consider that the Japanese almost do not eat sugar and sugar products, subjected to industrial processing. And indeed, the portions themselves are much smaller than other nations. Kies also did not consider countries that did not fit his theory, such as France, where people consumed a lot of saturated fat, and the percentage of incidence of cardiovascular disease was low. (Later this phenomenon would be called the French paradox.) Nevertheless, his ideas gained more and more popularity with the publication of many articles and books in which he talked about the relationship between saturated fats and degenerative heart diseases.

Presidential Influence

Kitty had a real talent for easily entering trust in people, including those in power. When Dwight Eisenhower suffered a massive heart attack in 1955, Paul Dudley White, the president's doctor's physician, listened to his advice. The next day, during the conference, White advised the public to consume less saturated fat and cholesterol to prevent heart disease, a recommendation he received from Keyes.

Using his influence and connections, Kies joined the American Association for the Study of Cardiovascular Diseases (ANA) nutrition committee. In 1961, the association published a report based on Kies's ideas, which advised patients at risk to reduce their intake of saturated fats. (It's awful to realize that ANA began to gain popularity in 1948 and received a $ 1.7 million donation from Procter & Gamble that same year, which turned it into a kind of debtor to Crisco manufacturers.)

In the same 1961, Times magazine placed on the cover of the new issue of Kitty in a white coat, calling him "the most influential nutrition expert in the 21st century."

In 1970, Keyes published A Study of Seven Countries, although there were six countries that he investigated, but this did not prevent the publication from producing a "burst bomb effect". Even today, you will find citations from there in more than a million scientific articles. Although Kies' research was never based on a causal relationship between saturated fats and heart disease, but only on associations, he was able to win the minds of ordinary people. And we continue to pay for it.

Thanks to Kies, the American medical community and modern media began to urge people to exclude the butter, lard and bacon that they had eaten for centuries from the diet and replace them with bread, pasta, margarine, low-fat dairy products and vegetable oil. This dietary change program was codified by the US government in the late 1970s and distributed throughout the world.

How Nutrition Guidelines Have Ruined A Nation's Health
In 1977, America released the first national dietary guide, forcing people to reduce fat intake. Moving away from the extremely popular diet of those years meant consuming more cereal products and less fat, while animal fats were replaced with refined vegetable oils.

According to a study by Zoe Harkombe, Ph.D., published in the Open Heart magazine , calls to remove fats from the American diet have never been scientifically based. Dr. Harkombe and her colleagues examined in detail the results of controlled randomized trials (RCTs) conducted during the introduction of the nutrition guidelines, a gold standard for scientific work available to US and UK controlled authorities. Six dietary studies included 2467 men. The results showed that the change in diet did not affect the percentage of deaths from common causes and slightly reduced the percentage of deaths from cardiovascular diseases.

Quoting Open Heart, "The recommendations were addressed to 276 million people after a second study of 2467 men. The percentage of deaths from common causes remained unchanged. Therefore, the RCT did not confirm the validity of a low-fat diet. "

Despite the lack of facts, the leadership was tough enough, urging people to reduce their total fat intake to 30%, in particular to limit saturated fats to just 10% of the total calorie share. War fats were in full swing and they still have not died out. In December 2015, the U.S. Department of Agriculture released a new nutrition guide and again raised concerns about saturated fats. Literally: "Saturated fat should account for less than 10% of calories per day".

For all these years, the government, with its recommendations, only exacerbated the problems that were supposed to solve it. No one knows exactly how many people died due to a low-fat diet, but I dare to assume that their number is hundreds of millions.

The Experiment With A Low-Fat Diet Ended In Complete Failure

Beginning in the 1950s, when Ansel Kies began popularizing a low-fat diet, Americans, followed by Europeans, honestly reduced the share of animal fat consumption. The peak of these changes occurred after the publication of the USDA nutrition guide in 1980 and the subsequent "reset" of the food industry, which began to produce low-fat foods, replacing healthy saturated fats such as butter and lard, with harmful transgenes - processed vegetable butter and a lot of refined sugar. (Food manufacturers needed to make their foods tastier despite the lack of a pleasant taste of butter and lard, so they added more and more sugar.)

Strict adherence to government regulations has led to a significant deterioration in the health of Americans. This is evidenced by the following statistics.

Diabetes

According to the U.S. Centers for Disease Control and Prevention, in 1978, 5.19 million Americans were diagnosed with diabetes. By 2013, this the figure increased to 22.3 million, i.e. more than four times in 35 years.

Obesity
According to the National Health and Nutrition Verification
Program, from 1976 to 1980, 16.4% of adults suffered from
moderate obesity (body mass index (BMI) above 30) or
extreme form (BMI above 35). The most recent data from the
Journal of the American Medical Association suggests that the
number of people with these two forms of obesity has
increased to 45.6% . Thus, in the 1970s, one in six was
overweight, and today, every second.
Oncology
Obesity increases the risk of cancer. In 1975, oncology was
detected in 400 people out of 100,000. According to
preliminary data, in 2016, 449 out of 100,000 received a terrible
diagnosis - a significant increase.
Heart Diseases
Heart disease is also associated with obesity. The mortality
rate from cardiovascular disease has declined compared to the
peak in the 1950s. This was largely due to the use of new
methods of treatment, but not the improvement of the health
of the nation.

The proportion of heart disease is high and continues to grow.
In 2010, approximately 36.9% of Americans had some form of
cardiovascular disease, and this is not the limit. A study
published in Circulation , a journal of the American
Association for the Study of Heart Diseases, states that by
2030, more than 40% of the US population will be living with
heart problems.

When you see the difference between the body's assimilation of sugars and fats, you can understand why all of these useless nutritional guidelines have been damaging the health of many nations for many years. Remember: your body receives more energy in the processing of fats than sugars. By consuming sugars and non-fiber carbohydrates, which quickly turn into glucose, you produce far more harmful free radicals than when you consume fats as the main fuel. Although free radicals perform a number of important health functions, with an excess of glucose and non-fiber carbohydrates, you are shifting the balance not in your favor. An imbalance leads to damage to tissues, protein, cell membrane, genetic disorders, which as a result causes inflammation and disease.

The war on saturated fats has affected not only our physical health. For decades, we have been advised by the government, doctors, and the leading media, arguing that you can be healthy and slim if you eat less - especially saturated fats - and move more. In reality, consuming foods high in fat and carbohydrates only complicates your task of losing weight. When we eat carbohydrates, the pancreas secretes insulin. And the more insulin in the blood, the more signals the body gives to store fat. Thus, following the dietary guidelines formally codified by the government in 1977, the Americans, and after them all the others, did everything to gain and maintain weight. Therefore, if you followed the advice of the USDA and leaned on bread, skimmed cereal and milk, and visited the gym a couple of times a week, and your extra pounds remained where they were, who is to blame? According to the same nutrition guidelines, you are to blame.

Perhaps you just did not try hard or did everything wrong. Complete demoralization. When I developed MMT and wrote this book, my main task was to show that it is in your power to lose weight and become healthy.

What Does Science Say?

Since Ansel Kies first published his observations, nothing much has changed. Avoid saturated fats, because they lead to increased cholesterol in the blood, clogged arteries and heart disease. The problem with this recommendation is that it was based on hypotheses (the worst), and these hypotheses have never been confirmed. In fact, decades of research studied the relationship between saturated fats and heart disease and found no justification.

Six major clinical trials of saturated fats were conducted, the purpose of which was to confirm their relationship with heart disease. In fact, none of them showed that reducing the intake of saturated fats prevents the occurrence of cardiovascular diseases and prolongs life, therefore, does not lead to a decrease in overall mortality.

A study in Oslo (1968) showed that consumption of a lower proportion of saturated and high amounts of polyunsaturated fats does not affect the level of sudden deaths.

A Los Angeles Veterans Health Survey (1969) showed that the percentage of sudden deaths and deaths from a heart attack among men who consumed large amounts of animal fats and men who consumed predominantly vegetable oils was approximately the same. But in the second group (a diet high in vegetable oil), the proportion of deaths from non-cardiac diseases, such as oncology, was higher.

The Minnesota Coronary Study (1968), conducted by the National Institutes of Health, showed that four years of consuming a low proportion of saturated and a high proportion of polyunsaturated fats did not lead to a reduction in cardiovascular disorders, deaths due to heart disease and general mortality.

A study of the Finnish Psychiatric Hospital (1968) showed a reduction in cardiovascular disease among men who consumed few saturated and many polyunsaturated fats, but this reduction was not observed among women.
A London study of soybean oil (1968) showed that the percentage of heart attacks among men who consumed low amounts of saturated fat and a lot of soybean oil was equal to the percentage of men on a traditional diet.

A multivariate prophylaxis study in the United States (1982), which compared mortality and nutritional preferences of 12,000 men, showed that those who consumed low saturated fat and cholesterol showed a slight decrease in coronary heart disease. This fact was widely publicized, in contrast to another circumstance: mortality from all causes was quite high.

As for our days, three meta-analyzes, which in total covered data on hundreds of thousands of people, showed that there was no difference in the percentage of risk of cardiovascular disease and heart attacks between groups on high-fat and low-fat diets. (Meta-analysis is a statistical scientific method of combining data from a certain amount of independent research.)

Some studies have shown that replacing saturated animal fats with plant-treated omega-6 fats has increased the risk of death among patients with heart disease. British Medical Journal 2013 published the results of a scientific test involving 458 men with heart problems. Men were divided into two groups. The first group consumed a reduced proportion of saturated fats (less than 10% of the total energy share) and a larger volume of omega-6 safflower oils (15% of the total energy share). The second control group continued to eat as they wanted. As a result, after 39 months: in the first group that consumed omega-6 linoleic acid, the risk of death from cardiovascular disease during the study increased by 17% compared with 11% in the second control group; in the omega-6 group, the risk of dying from all causes also increased.

Another test, published in the British Medical Journal in 2013, found that replacing saturated animal fats with processed vegetable fats enriched with omega-6 leads to an increased risk of death among patients with heart disease.

The Truth About Saturated Fats

The bias against saturated fats is largely due to their effect on cholesterol in the form of low density lipoproteins (LDL cholesterol), which is also called "bad" cholesterol. It is important to understand that both the terms "LDL" and "HDL" refer to lipoproteins - simple proteins that contain cholesterol.

LDL is low density lipoprotein, and HDL is high density lipoprotein. HDL cholesterol is associated with a lower risk of heart disease. This is why measuring total cholesterol is useless when you want to know the risks you are exposed to. In fact, if the total level of cholesterol in the blood is high due to the large amount of HDL, this does not indicate an increased risk of heart disease, but rather the opposite. Saturated fats, as it turned out, increase the level of protective HDL, reducing the proportion of LDL. The latter is also not always "bad", because it is divided into several types:
Small dense LDL cholesterol - "bad";
Large light LDL cholesterol is "good."

Synthetic trans fats increase the level of small dense LDL cholesterol in the blood, and saturated fats lead to an increase in the proportion of large lungs - "useful" - LDL.

Large light LDL particles are absolutely safe for the heart. But small, dense LDL particles easily penetrate the walls of arteries and can cause them to become clogged.

In people with high levels of low dense LDL cholesterol, the risk of heart disease is three times higher than in people with high levels of high low LDL cholesterol. And here is another fact that will surprise you greatly: consumption of saturated fats can turn small dense LDL in your body into "good" big lungs! It's important to remember: studies have shown that the number of small dense LDL particles increases when you eat refined sugar and carbohydrates, such as bread and donuts, or drink soda.

Together, refined sugar and carbohydrates do much more harm to the body than saturated fats. With all of the above, now you understand how much saturated fats are important for maintaining health and preventing disease. In fact, they participate in a number of important body processes, such as the provision of "building bricks" for cell membranes, hormones and hormone-like substances; absorption of minerals, for example calcium; supplying the body with fat-soluble vitamins A, D, E, K; conversion of carotene to vitamin A; lowering blood cholesterol (palmitic and stearic acid); virus control (acrylic acid); supplying the brain with energy in the process of converting fats into ketones; the appearance of a feeling of satiety and satisfaction - that is, most likely, you will not want to have a bite to eat products that have undergone industrial processing, which taste good but are not at all useful; modulation of genetic regulation and prevention of oncological diseases (butyric acid); an increase in LDL, mainly large and light particles, which do not lead to cardiovascular disease; an increase in the level of HDL that can compensate for any increase in the proportion of LDL; energy supply to mitochondria and the production of fewer free radicals than in the processing of carbohydrates.

The study clearly showed that saturated fats benefit our body. Many of us need to significantly increase the proportion of healthy fats in the diet. This includes not only saturated fats, but also monounsaturated (avocados and some nuts) and omega-3 fatty acids. It is also necessary to reduce the proportion of refined vegetable oils, even those that contain omega-6 (nuts and seeds).

If you're afraid you don't remember so much information, just follow one simple rule:
To maintain health, eat "live" foods - a lot of saturated fats and nothing processed, especially exclude refined vegetable oils.

Chapter 5 - Why Do You Need Mitochondrial Metabolic Therapy (MMT)?

Whether you are faced with serious health problems or simply want to "recharge" your body, this chapter is for you.

Why Exactly MMT?

As I said, the proper functioning of mitochondria is the key to your health. Each cell of the body contains from 80 to 2000 mitochondria, and they generate approximately 90% of the energy that allows you to live and be healthy. When mitochondrial function is disrupted, it's easy if you are sitting on a typical low-fat, high-carb diet with a high proportion of products that have undergone industrial processing - in turn, the normal metabolic signaling process is disrupted, cellular and mitochondrial DNA are affected, and a defect in the system of restoring other types of damage occurs, for example, as a result of environmental radiation.

In order for the body to be able to prevent the disease or fight cancer and other diseases, you must take special care of mitochondria. And the main way to optimize, restore and regenerate mitochondria is to provide them with the best fuel. This is why mitochondrial metabolic therapy is needed.

MMT does not offer you ways to control the symptoms of chronic diseases, it heals the root cause of their occurrence, as well as the cause of aging - the presence or absence of mitochondrial integrity.

The integrity of mitochondria is the key to youth!

The Difference Between MMT And The Atkins And Paleo Diets

I consider MMT to be the best nutritional scheme for optimizing mitochondrial function, but there are many other popular diets, in some respects similar to MMT. Although there are key differences between them. These diets are:

• Atkins Diet . A pioneer in nutrition, Dr. Robert Atkins, said in the 1970s that consuming a lot of carbohydrates is unhealthy. His first book, The Atkins Dietary Revolution, sold 15 million copies, and with its help, more than 30 million people are on a low-carb diet. Pay attention to the word "low-carb ", he urged to pay attention to the reduction of carbohydrates, and not burning fat.

Atkins introduced the term "ketosis" to the general public, but since the word is similar to the word "ketoacidosis," a deadly condition that occurs with type 1 diabetes, he quickly turned people's attention to fats as the main sources of energy. The main pests on our table were declared bread and pasta. Atkins was close to developing the perfect diet. Of course, he made a coup, especially in the minds of ordinary people. His role in education is undeniable. But at the same time in his diet, there were several drawbacks.

The main thing is to reduce weight. The Atkins diet has gained great popularity because its main promise was weight loss, quick and effortless. Although losing weight can have a positive effect on your health, weight loss (especially fat) is just a side effect of MMT. Of course, many will be happy with such a side effect, but the real goals of MMT are to restore metabolism at the cellular level, prevent the development of common chronic diseases and inhibit the aging process - a much more ambitious task than just trying to get into tight jeans again.

Too much protein. Since the war on fats was in full swing, the Atkins diet turned into a dangerous fad, and ketosis was seen as an abnormal and undesirable metabolic state. Although Atkins advised consuming leafy green vegetables, many of his followers leaned too much on protein to replace the calories that would otherwise come from carbohydrates. As a result, a stereotype arose that people on the Atkins diet ate too much fried meat, eggs, cheese, and bacon.

I will explain why a high-protein diet is much more dangerous than a high-carb diet. To date, the average European consumes too much protein. It was to solve this problem that MMT was developed by me.

Zero attention to product quality. Perhaps the most important thing Atkins did not tell his followers is the need to avoid low-quality foods, and it doesn't matter if it's beef, pasteurized dairy products or refined vegetable oil. Paying great attention to macronutrients (a term that encompasses a wide range of nutrients such as carbohydrates, fats and proteins) is correct, but some foods containing macronutrients alone are dangerous to health. As a result, the Atkins diet provoked inflammation and crippled mitochondria. In addition, many products recommended by the doctor - and these are bars and cocktails with high content of artificial sweeteners - belonged to the category of "chemical" food.

Will or will not your body burn fat. Although the diet was low-carb, many who ate according to Atkins continued to consume a lot of protein, making it harder for the body to switch to burning fat. This process, which takes weeks, if not months, requires constant monitoring of glucose and ketone levels to really make sure that your body is rebuilt to burn fat. (A little later I will talk about this process in more detail.)

The Paleo diet was based on the eating habits of our ancestors of the Paleolithic era, which consumed mainly vegetables, fruits, nuts, roots and meat. The Paleo diet called for the abandonment of cereals and legumes but did not impose any restrictions on high-carb vegetables, fruits, and sugars, such as honey or coconut sugar.

The popularity of the Paleo diet is well founded. It brings us back to the roots, offering us to eat fresh, wholesome, unprocessed "live" food, and this is the main step towards optimizing our health and may well suit each of us. Although the Paleo diet is a healthy eating plan and a good substitute for a standard diet, it has a number of disadvantages that make it far from ideal.

Too much protein. Proteins freely replaced carbohydrates as healthier. The Paleo diet called for consuming 38% of proteins and 39% of fats but there are too many proteins to maintain a healthy diet and carbohydrates are simply not enough. As I will tell you later, a protein level of about 10% in the process of nutritious ketosis is considered optimal. This percentage may be higher, especially for those who are at the age of the peak of reproductive functions or in good physical shape but maintaining a high level of protein for a long time is considered undesirable.

No caution for seafood. The Paleo diet involves the regular use of large quantities of fish and seafood. This is justified, because docosahexaenoic acid (DHA) is a fatty acid of the class omega-3, which is found in fish, is one of the main nutrients for maintaining good health. But there is an important caveat: as a result of environmental pollution and emissions, the atmosphere of toxic substances, including Mercury, polychlorinated biphenyls (PCBs) and dioxins, it is difficult to find environmentally friendly seafood. That's why I recommend eating fish that is rich in healthy fats and has been minimally contaminated.

Too Much Starch And Sugar (Pure Carbohydrates)
Although sweet potatoes and fruits are two of the most popular Paleo diet foods, they are high-grade foods, they can increase blood glucose and trigger an insulin reaction, especially if you are looking for a way to rebuild your body to burn fat. This is completely useless if you have already been rebuilt and your body uses fats rather than carbohydrates as its main fuel. The main goal of MMT is to lower blood glucose and, accordingly, insulin in order to regulate insulin resistance.

To some extent, MMT can be considered as a modified Paleo diet: it is the consumption of high-grade food, no grains, a lot of attention to the quality of products, the proportion of non-fiber carbohydrates - about 50 grams per day (or less), the rejection of natural sugars, such as dates (except for those sweeteners, about which will be discussed later).

The problem is clear. On the one hand, mitochondria play a big role maintaining overall health, they synthesize ATP and control apoptosis (a program of cell death), as well as autophagy and mitophagy, which remove unhealthy cells and mitochondria before they contribute to the development of chronic diseases. On the other hand, mitochondria are the basis for the formation of ROS and damage to free radicals, since they contain two cell membranes, internal and external, both very fragile.

Ketones Are An Ideal Fuel For Brain Cells

The question is to produce ATP as efficiently as possible in order to optimize health and increase life expectancy, while avoiding the problems that arise when consuming foods that contribute to the production of excess free radicals in the metabolic process.

Ketones produce far less free radicals as an energy source than sugar. They simply serve as a cleaner fuel, which means they cause less oxidative damage - one of the main reasons why diets based on burning fat, including MMT, are so effective.

Reducing the proportion of damage due to oxidation occurs with a low level of glucose in the blood. This was proved by Dr. Seyfried in a work on the glycemic ketone index. This is why tracking blood sugar levels is an integral part of MMT.

Additional Benefits Of Mitochondrial Metabolic Therapy

In addition to filling your body with cleaner fuel and limiting the production of ROS, MMT has many other physiological advantages. If you look objectively, you will see that following such a diet is the best thing you can do for your health. Consider the pros.

Clarity Of Mind

Your brain cannot function properly without healthy fats. Since the brain is 60% fat, healthy fats, which make up biologically resistant cell membranes, are essential for optimal mental function. In contrast, too strong a passion for cereals and sugar leads to neural disorders and damage, partly as a result of blocking the ability of insulin to regulate normal cellular activity. The relationship between sugar and Alzheimer's was first discovered in 2005, when the disease was considered type 3 diabetes. Earlier studies have also shown that diabetics double the risk of developing Alzheimer's disease. Now it is not surprising that MMT, which will facilitate the reconfiguration of your body to burn fat, temporarily abandoning almost all high-carb foods in the diet, contributes to clarity of mind. By improving your brain today, you will protect yourself from dementia tomorrow.

I would not have written this book so fast if it were not for MMT and its amazing effect on the brain. I felt the power of inspiration and active mental work on myself, and I needed Google Keep, an application for creating notes on my computer, to quickly and easily write down new ideas and thoughts, and then not get lost in them.

No Cravings To Eat

Industrial food with all its chemical additives, sugar, refined oils and carbohydrates is highly addictive. This has been confirmed by a number of studies and scientific papers. It's no coincidence. The food industry employs a team of scientists who work to improve the taste of chemical foods. Thus, they increase the sense of traction, and you want to eat more and more, even when the body no longer needs it.

Sugar turns you into a hamster that eats, eats and eats. When sugar is the main fuel for the body, metabolic pathways are activated, and this causes a desire to eat, due to the fact that a few hours without sugar leads to a decrease in its level in the blood.

Fats, in turn, cause a feeling of fullness, which means that the stomach is full and you are not drawn to the refrigerator. When fats become the main fuel of the body, you get access to tens of thousands of calories, which are stored in the fat of your own body, calories that remain out of work when the body burns mainly sugar. As a result, you will go about your business and not even think about food for a long time. Any craving will pass when your body begins to "refuel" with fatty fuel.

One "but": if you suddenly notice that you want to eat fats, you have previously consumed them in insufficient quantities. This is one of the reasons why I love fat bombs (fat bombs) - a delicious treat, mainly consisting of coconut oil or other healthy fats - they are affordable and very tasty. One, two - and a couple of teaspoons of fat in your stomach.

Anti-Cancer Strategy

In recent years, scientists have found that the cause of oncology is not at all genetic mutations. Now we know that the root cause is damage to the mitochondria. Mitochondrial dysfunctions generate reactive oxygen species, which, in turn, disrupting the respiratory process, lead to DNA mutations. ROS damage mitochondria and their respiratory process. Thus, a vicious cycle arises.

It took decades for medicine to come to this. In 1924, Otto Warburg, who received the Nobel Prize in Physiology or Medicine in 1931, made a discovery - the so-called Warburg Effect, according to which the energy metabolism of cancer cells is fundamentally different from healthy cells. The Warburg effect shows that most mitochondria in cancer cells are dysfunctional and cannot use oxygen to burn fuel - they do not have metabolic flexibility for the exchange of fats. As a result, they live off by fermenting a growing proportion of glucose in the cytoplasm (instead of oxidizing it in the mitochondria), and this is an ineffective way of generating energy, called lactic acid fermentation.

Scientists have proven that cancer is not a genetic mutation, but the result of mitochondrial damage! Dr. Thomas N. Seyfried, a world-famous researcher on the relationship between metabolism and disease, and the author of the 2012 bestselling book Cancer as a Metabolic Disease, was able to find new evidence to refute the theory of cancer as a result of genetic changes. He identified forms of cancer that do not have genetic mutations, but receive energy in the process of fermentation, not respiration. In addition, there are carcinogens, such as arsenic and asbestos, which do not directly lead the occurrence of genetic mutations. Rather, they harm the respiratory function of mitochondria, which further causes the Warburg effect and cancer.

Seyfried found that the growth of cancer cells stops when the nucleus of the tumor cell is transferred to a normal cell with healthy mitochondria. The abnormal growth and metastases of breast cancer cells also stop when the mitochondria of the cancer cells are replaced by healthy mitochondria, even while maintaining the tumor cell nuclei.

This and other studies show that oncology is not a genetic disease. From the above it follows that when you refuse industrial products, sugar, grains and a large proportion of pure carbohydrates, you expose the cancer cells to great stress, depriving them of their main metabolic fuel.

Therefore, I believe that MMT is one of the most powerful cancer prevention strategies today, as it optimizes mitochondrial function and, therefore, makes them more resilient. The risk of genetic mutations that can lead to a terrible disease is sharply reduced.

MMT has several advantages if you are struggling with cancer. By reprogramming the body to burn ketones, you deprive the main fuel of the tumor cells, creating additional stress for them. At the same time, healthy cells receive a cleaner and higher quality fuel, reducing the proportion of oxidation, preserving antioxidants and optimizing the functioning of mitochondria. Healthy cells are in favorable conditions, and cancer cells are forced to fight for life.

Microbiome Changes

According to modern research, the human body contains about 30 trillion bacteria and 1 quadrillion viruses (bacteriophages). In other words, you and I are walking microbial colonies. These microorganisms perform a number of functions, including the following:

- Helping us digest food.
- Regulate the intestinal nervous system responsible for the digestive tract.
- Regulate immune resistance.
- They help to modulate aspects of inflammatory processes.
- They play an important role in maintaining the health of the brain and the entire mental system, since the intestines and brain are connected to each other.

Scientists have found that a microbial can quickly change for the better and for the worse depending on factors (diet, lifestyle, and chemical effects) - simple drugs and antibiotics, including those found in food, especially meat.

MMT nutrition plan regulates, changes and improves the intestinal microflora. It helps reduce the negative effects on the microbial by eliminating sugars, industrial foods and artificial sweeteners.

Chapter 6 - Weight Loss Without Loss

When the body burns glucose as the main fuel, access to the fats of your body and the process of burning them are difficult. In the presence of existing carbohydrates, the liver slows down the process of burning fat, because you do not follow the "saturated - starving" diet. Excess glucose is deposited in the form of fat, unlike ketones, which, not being absorbed by cells, are excreted in the urine.

Fat cells produce their own hormones, including leptin. If you constantly consume large amounts of sugar and store fat, leptin levels increase and its receptors become less sensitive. Restoring optimal leptin levels becomes more difficult. Therefore, when glucose is the main fuel of your body, fat cells become prisoners of the vicious cycle: fat continues to be deposited, and it becomes almost impossible to burn it.

When you eat a lot of sugar, fat is not processed into energy, but stored in your body.

Hormones and the relationship between them play an important role in controlling weight and in your desire to eat and what exactly to eat, because these hormones are determined by the food you consume.

This is the main principle of MMT. She perceives food as a way of forming the level of hormones - leptin and insulin - affecting body weight and forcing him to burn fat, and not put off. In addition, therapy eliminates the sources of sugars from your diet, breaking the vicious cycle. The body is released from excess weight. At the same time, you do not feel hunger and craving to eat, as is often the case with most diets for weight loss.

Much More Energy

MMT heals existing mitochondria and stimulates the emergence of new ones. Since mitochondria are the main sources of energy, MMT leads to its perceptible surge due to the fact that the body begins to produce less destructive ROS (because it metabolizes ketone bodies instead of sugar), you will need less cellular energy to remove bad free radicals - the proportion of pure energy in MMT increases.

Hypersensitivity To Insulin

Any full meal or snack high in pure carbohydrates leads to a sharp increase in blood sugar. To fix this, your pancreas begins to produce insulin, which, in turn, lowers blood sugar to normal, as excess glucose poisons the cells. Insulin also lowers blood sugar by inhibiting liver glucose production (gluconeogenesis).

Unfortunately, if you constantly consume large amounts of sugar and cereals, respectively, high blood sugar levels remain, and your insulin receptors gradually become "desensitized" to insulin, requiring more and more for the process. This applies to the field of insulin resistance. Today, approximately 45% of the inhabitants of developed countries have some form of insulin resistance, and this figure will only increase over time.

Since MMT does not mean eating foods that your body can easily turn into glucose, such as cereals, sugar, and foods with a high proportion of pure carbohydrates, your blood sugar remains low, as are your insulin levels. Lowering your sugar and insulin levels allows your insulin receptors to restore their own sensitivity.

Reduce Inflammation

Sugar adds fuel to the fire of your inflammatory processes, as it is dirty fuel. Nature did not create it as our main source of energy. By burning sugar, we produce 30–40% more ROS than by burning fat.

Omega-6 oils, especially those that are highly refined and easily oxidized , provoke inflammation. With MMT, you limit your intake of bad fats and get all the essentials from oil-rich foods. And it will be healthy oils! By increasing the proportion of omega-3 fatty acids in your diet, you will thereby balance the proportion of omega-6 to omega-3, which is important for maintaining health. In addition, saturated fats are not as easily oxidizable as oils, because they do not have double bonds that can be damaged during the oxidation process. MMT encourages you to use the right sources of healthy saturated and monounsaturated fats, as well as lower your intake of omega-6 fatty acids. Now it is not surprising that, according to studies, low-carb diets reduce the amount of systemic inflammation.

Self-Eating: Autophagy And Mitophagy

The term "autophagy" literally translates as "self-eating." These are processes, as a result of which your body is cleansed of accumulated debris, such as toxins, and processes damaged cell components. Autophagy occurs inside the mitochondria. When mitochondria is destroyed and disposed of, it is called mitophagy.

Both processes are critical to maintaining a healthy body. In 2016, Yoshinori Osumi, a scientist who discovered autophagy mechanisms, received the Nobel Prize in physiology or medicine. When autophagy and mitophagy are restrained as a result of poor nutrition, the presence of excess ROS and multiple inflammatory processes, damaged mitochondria are retained in the cells, releasing molecules that provoke inflammation and accelerate the aging of the body. Thus, autophagy and mitophagy play a very important role. They control inflammation in the human body and slow down aging.

For the most part, these processes occur under the mechanistic goal of rapamycin (in mammals), a regulator of metabolic signaling pathways. When mTOR is activated, growth and regeneration processes are started, including cellular level. MMT inhibits the containment (down regulation) of these mTOR signaling pathways, thereby stimulating autophagy and mitophagy.

Mitochondrial Biogenesis (The Formation Of New Mitochondria)

Biogenesis is the process of division, as a result of which new healthy mitochondria is born. When we talk about maintaining optimal biological functions of the body and feeling good, the healthier your mitochondria are, the better.

Studies have shown that switching to a fat burning diet activates mitochondrial biogenesis, at least in rodents. With this kind of nutrition, mitochondria are not exclusively occupied with the fight against free radicals (since fat burning produces much less harmful reactive oxygen particles than burning sugar). The positive effect is that mitochondria have much more energy for the formation of new healthy mitochondria. As a result, your mitochondria are full of vitality!

The Effect Of Ketones

When I say that with MMT you "burn fat", it means that you burn ketones or ketone bodies. Ketones and ketone bodies are interchangeable, and often one replaces the other. In this book, I will talk specifically about ketones.

Ketones are water-soluble energy molecules that are synthesized by liver mitochondria from dietary or stored fats and are used by the body as an alternative to glucose fuel. Since ketones dissolve in water, they don't need protein to travel through the bloodstream. They easily penetrate cell membranes and even cross the homoencephalic barrier.

Our brain does not use sugar at all as energy, as is commonly thought, but ketones. In fact, ketones are excellent biological adaptants that supply vital fuel to the brain and body when consuming scarce food. Without ketones in case of hunger, you would not have lived for several days. It used to be that the brain uses only sugar as a fuel, even today many experts continue to believe this. The deceitful theory was refuted by the late George Cahill exactly 50 years ago. In fact, your body delivers fuel to the brain in a special way, which consumes up to 20% of all calories. The ability of the brain to adapt to ketone metabolism helps a person survive without food for several weeks to a month.

The longest fasting period in history was 1 year and 17 days. Only thanks to ketones was it possible to accomplish such a feat. Ketones are an important component of MMT, their presence shows that you burn fats, not sugar, as the main fuel. There are three types of ketones.

Acetoacetate is a precursor to two other forms of ketones. It is excreted in the urine. Beta-hydroxybutyrate (BOMC) are the most numerous ketones that circulate with the blood and give energy. Acetone - is released during exhalation.

Are Ketones Geniuses Or Villains?

Unfortunately, today among not only ordinary people, but even some experts there is confusion regarding ketones. It is associated with the presence of a significant difference between nutritional ketosis and diabetic ketoacidosis. Although both of these words have the prefix "keto," they denote two different metabolic states.

Nutrient ketosis - the initial stage in the transition to fat burning. This is a favorable way to create an environment that helps you stay healthy and young. With nutritional ketosis, the level of ketones in the blood usually ranges from 0.5–3 mmol / L and rarely exceeds 6–8 mmol / L. Blood sugar levels also drop to an optimal level of 70 mg / dl or less.

Ketoacidosis, on the other hand, is an extremely dangerous symptom of uncontrolled diabetes, which, if untreated, can lead to death. Ketone levels in diabetic ketoacidosis are usually greater than 20 mmol / L. The real danger of diabetic ketoacidosis is a very high blood sugar level of 250 mg / dl, and sometimes this figure exceeds 400 mg / dl! As a result, severe metabolic acidosis and severe dehydration occur, requiring intensive medical intervention.

Ketoacidosis occurs in type 1 diabetes due to low insulin levels. Since the body needs insulin to suppress the production of glucose by the liver, it continues to be produced even when you are not eating. A high glucose level should "turn off" the production of ketones, but at the same time, the lack of insulin is characterized by the absence of a signal to stop the process. If there is a lot of glucose in the body, the brain does not use ketones as fuel. They accumulate and provoke metabolic acidosis. On the other hand, with nutritious ketosis, if you have not starved for a long time, enough insulin accumulates in the body to suppress the production of glucose by the liver. Glucose drops stay low when you reduce your carbohydrate intake, and the brain begins to burn ketones.

Thus, the deadly metabolic state associated with diabetic ketoacidosis is the effect of the simultaneous exposure to very high levels of ketones, high glucose and dehydration. Such a condition cannot occur with nutritious ketosis, but this is precisely the stumbling block for many of today's doctors with outdated views.

Dr. Atkins was the first to introduce ketosis to the general public as the desired effect of consuming less carbohydrates, but the term "nutritional ketosis," alas, does not yet exist. Due to confusion and demonization of fats, Atkins practically refused to use this term in his book, paying much attention not to the benefits of burning fat, but to the carbohydrate aspect.

Subsequent studies (Dr. Atkins died in 2004) revealed a difference in the effects of healthy and unhealthy fats on the body. Thank God, in the 21st century there are many published scientific papers confirming the metabolic benefits of nutritious ketosis. These works, together with the testimonies of people who have discovered the benefits that have been identified, little by little clarify the situation, allowing health professionals and ordinary doctors, who had previously ignored nutrition, to start using diets in their practice.

Why Do We Need Ketones?

Ketones were discovered in the late 1800s. They were found in the urine of patients with uncontrolled diabetes. After several decades, scientists have identified positive aspects of ketone production. If the proportion of carbohydrates received with food is small or zero even after a few days, your body begins to convert fats to ketones. This metabolic flexibility is the main reason why humanity is still alive. It helps us adapt to different food sources. Besides the ability to survive the hungry years, ketones have a huge positive effect on our health.

When cells burn ketones as their primary fuel, the body produces less ROS than when glucose is burned. In fact, ketones are a "cleaner" source of energy than glucose, which means they do much less harm to mitochondria. If you are tuned to burning fat (and ketones), your body's share of the sugar that feeds the cancer cells is reduced. In addition, the amount of ROS that the cells are exposed to is reduced. The risk of cancer falls.

The most numerous ketones, beta-hydroxybutyrate, perform a number of different signaling functions that affect gene expression. Ketones play an important role in reducing inflammatory processes by reducing (down-regulating) the number of cytokines that cause inflammation and increasing the number (up-regulation) of cytokines, which are suppressive.

Ketones are similar in structure to branched chain amino acids (B C A A). Nevertheless, they are preferable for the body than BCAAs. Ketones have a gentle protein effect that allows you to consume less protein, while maintaining and even building muscle mass. In addition, BCAAs are an effective stimulus for mTOR molecular signaling pathways, a very important metabolic pathway, which in the case of illness (including oncology) is in a state of hyperactivity. By supporting nutritional ketosis, you are holding back mTOR. The decrease in activity in this case is associated with health and life expectancy. However, mTOR plays an important role, especially for young people, as a powerful stimulator of protein synthesis in muscles. Many athletes and bodybuilders purposefully activate these paths, thereby reducing life expectancy.

Studies show that ketones perform a number of important protective functions of brain cells, which are exposed to hydrogen peroxide, which is usually found in the brain of people suffering from neurodegenerative diseases, such as dementia and Alzheimer's disease. With increasing levels of iron, hydrogen peroxide turns into dangerous hydroxyl free radicals. Thus, you can get the maximum benefit from ketones with an optimal level of iron.

Ketones up-regulate (enhance) the biogenesis of mitochondria in the brain. This means that by increasing the number of mitochondria, they help your body produce more energy. There is a funny observation: people during hunger or when switching to a low-carb diet experience mild euphoria. Thus, ketones are the key to a good mood.

Despite the advantages, the main objective of MMT is not to produce enough ketones for nutrient ketosis. Our main goal is to start eating healthy foods and switch to fat burning. That's why I will never call MMT the "ketogenic diet", a term that describes a similar high-fat, low-carb diet. Such diets are built solely on how to produce the highest possible number of ketones. This does not suit us. As I already said, the ultimate goal of MMT is to optimize the functioning of mitochondria, to reduce the damage caused to the body by free radicals, and to influence the root cause of the disease. Ketones in this case are not a goal, but a means.

Improved Quality Of Life And Survival Of Children With Brain Cancer

Miriam Kalamian has the richest experience in applying MMT principles for cancer treatment. She helped me with the editing of this book, and I asked her to share with readers the story of her son, who prompted Miriam to help cancer patients.

"When my dear son Ruffy was four years old, doctors discovered a brain tumor in him. Confused, my husband and I immediately agreed to standard treatment: 14 months of weekly treatments combined with chemotherapeutic drugs. When the treatment failed, Raffi was prescribed even less effective therapy. After a year and a half, he underwent several complex operations due to progressive hydrocephalus manifestations of side effects from drugs used previously. The treatment suffered more and more failures. It became clear that our baby is losing a ruthless struggle with the disease. At seven, he began to receive palliative care. The story could have ended on this, if one night I didn't sit down to look for information about a drug that my son accepted and didn't stumble upon the revolutionary research of Dr. Thomas Seyfried. According to his theory, cancer is mainly a metabolic disease, which should be treated with a diet. So is it possible to save Ruffy without toxic pills?

I was extremely excited, and, as it turned out, there were many difficulties ahead of us. Firstly, I did not have a specialty nutritionist. Secondly , there was no such precedent for a high-fat, low-carb diet to be used as cancer therapy. Fortunately, the doctors at John Hopkins Hospital, who have extensive experience using such a diet to treat childhood epilepsy, have released a new book that suggests that a ketogenic diet helps people with brain cancer.

Then, on the Charlie Foundation website, I met my parents, who were already versed in all these ketone issues , which helped me a lot. Of course, I could not have traveled such a long and difficult path without the support of the oncologist and pediatrician Raffi. Thanks to them, we were able to overcome the fears and obstacles that leading experts put before us.

In the spring of 2007, my husband and I put Raffi on a ketogenic diet, armed with those bits of information that we had. Following the regimen designed for patients with epilepsy, I decided to start with fasting. It was a hard (mentally and physically) first day. Thank God , the metabolism in children is much more flexible than in adults, so Raffy quickly switched to ketones and fats. In fact, the beginning was no worse than the many days during which Raffy had to experience the gastrointestinal side effect of the drugs.

Surprisingly, the symptoms of the disease immediately subsided. Ruffy had more strength, a clearer mind and even a little better vision, which his tumor deprived. We knew we were on the right track! It took a certain amount of time and effort to achieve tangible success. We were generously rewarded. Three short months after starting the diet, MRI showed slight compression tumor mass.

It was like a shock to me. After all, no one knows about this miraculous treatment. A ketogenic diet is nothing more than a mixture of familiar foods. Why is it so stubbornly rejected by official medicine and society?

Ruffy's success gave me the urge to talk about this diet (as a supplement, not a replacement for the main treatment). After a couple of weeks, I signed up for higher nutrition courses, believing that one day I could share my knowledge with people and offer them a diet that can not only improve the quality of life, but, possibly, extend it.

Unfortunately, Ruffy could not defeat the disease, we learned too late about the ketogenic diet. Six years that he spent on a ketogenic diet, our family caught moments of happiness. We spent five amazing months in a camp on the Bach Peninsula. The sun, the beach, and doing nothing were much better than a hospital bed. All this, as well as the sense of confidence and control that the diet gave, inspired me to help others. The memory of Ruffy is another important incentive.

I started official practice in 2010. Since then, I have helped hundreds of cancer patients transition to a therapeutic diet. Although many people have experienced what their oncologists have called the "amazing response to treatment," the diet remains extremely unpopular and unclaimed in a world where scientists are proud to invent new treatments and millions continue to die from a terrible disease. I sincerely believe in the effectiveness of the ketone diet, and that is why I gladly agreed to share my personal experience with the readers of this wonderful book that illuminates our path to good health. "

Chapter 7 - Recipes

Ketogenic Breakfast

Calories: 106.2 kcal | Protein: 10.4 grams | Fat: 6.6 grams | Carbohydrates: 1.3 grams

Ingredients for one person:

1 egg | 1 tbsp cream cheese with 0.2% FiT | 1 tbsp almond flour | 1 splash of sweetener | 1 pinch of cinnamon ground | 1 pinch of Himalayan salt

Preparation:

1.   Beat the egg until well frothy with the whisk and stir until smooth with the cream cheese.
2.   Work in the almond flour and season with sweetener, cinnamon, and salt.
3.   Bake in a nonstick pan to a pancake.
4.   If necessary, sprinkle with a little streuxylitol.

Calories: 127.4 kcal | Protein: 7.8 grams | Fat: 5.4 grams | Carbohydrates: 11.9 grams

Ingredients for one person:

150 grams of yogurt | Juice, and attrition of half an organic lime | 1 splash of sweetener | 60 grams of berry mix fresh or TK | 1 teaspoon lemon balm chopped

Preparation:

1.   Stir the yogurt with the juice and the grated lime and season with sweetener.
2.   Carefully fold in the berries and garnish with the lemon balm.
3.   If you'd rather enjoy a smoothie for breakfast, just put all the ingredients in the blender and process them into a creamy shake.
4.   On hot days, you can also add some ice cubes to the blender and in a flash, you can make a kind of keto frozen yogurt.

Calories: 290 kcal | Protein: 24.6 grams | Fat: 20.8 grams | Carbohydrates: 1.1 grams

Ingredients for one person:

2 eggs | 1/2 teaspoon dill chopped | 1 pinch of cream horseradish | 1/2 teaspoon butter |1 pinch of Himalayan salt | white pepper | 80 grams of smoked salmon

Preparation:

1.   Stir the eggs with the dill and the horseradish and season with salt and pepper.

2.   Beware, the smoked salmon itself is usually salty enough.

3.   In a pan with hot butter, the egg to a scrambled eggs process and just before the end of the smoked salmon cut into strips.

4.   You can also sprinkle the scrambled eggs with fresh chives or finely chopped chili.

Calories: 147.2 kcal | Protein: 9.2 grams | Fat: 11.6 grams | Carbohydrates: 1.5 grams

Ingredients for one person:

1 egg | 2 tbsp. Curd | 1 pinch of Himalayan salt | white pepper | 1/2 teaspoon sesame black

Preparation:

1.   Separate the egg and process the egg whites into stiff snow.

2.   Smooth the yolk with the quark and season with salt and pepper.

3.   Carefully fold in the egg whites.

4.   Layout a baking tray with baking paper and heat the oven to 180 ° (top/bottom heat).

5.   Put a heap on the baking paper and sprinkle with black sesame seeds.

6.   Bake the cloud bread for 8 minutes.

Calories: 194.5 kcal | Protein: 13.6 grams | Fat: 14.5 grams | Carbohydrates: 2.4 grams

Ingredients for one person:

2 eggs | 1/2 teaspoon butter | 1 tomato | 1 tsp chives cut into rolls | 1 pinch of Himalayan salt | pepper from the grinder

Preparation:

1.   Whisk the eggs well with the whisk.
2.   Free the tomato from the core and cut into small cubes.
3.   Sauté them in the butter for about 2 minutes and lightly salt and pepper.
4.   Add the egg and let it stand slowly in a low flame.
5.   Tear with a spatula and sprinkle generously with chives before serving.

Calories: 37.6 kcal | Protein: 6.4 grams | Fat: 0.4 grams | Carbohydrates: 2.1 grams

Ingredients for one person:

150 ml vegetable broth | 1/2 cm ginger | 5 cm lemongrass | 1 red chilli | 2 shrimp peeled and cleaned | 20 grams of konjac rice | 1 tbsp coriander roughly chopped | Soy sauce bright | Fish sauce | 5 grams of bean sprouts

Preparation:

1.   Peel the ginger and cut into thin slices.
2.   Cut the lemongrass into 1 cm pieces and bring to the boil.
3.   Finely chop the chili and add.
4.   Rinse the konjac rice and cook in the broth for 3 minutes.
5.   Cut the prawns into small pieces and also cook in the soup.
6.   Season with soy sauce and fish sauce, cook for another minute, then remove from heat, stir in the bean sprouts and serve.
7.   Sprinkle generously with cilantro and enjoy.

Calories: 104.6 kcal | Protein: 14.5 grams | Fat: 2.6 grams | Carbohydrates: 5.8 grams

Ingredients for one person:

130 grams of cottage cheese 10% fat | 1 red chilli | 1 pinch of grated ginger | some abrasion of a bio lime | 1/2 teaspoon chopped chili | 1 pinch of Himalayan salt

Preparation:

1.   Stir the quark with the finely chopped chili and mix with the ginger and the grated lime.

2.   Season salt with Himalaya salt and sprinkle with chervil.

3.   The spicy quark is a great alternative for those who do not like to have a sweet breakfast.

4.   If you like the quark nice and sharp, it is best to let it through overnight or for at least 30 minutes.

Calories: 316 kcal | Protein: 29.5 grams | Fat: 21.6 grams | Carbohydrates: 0.9 grams

Ingredients for one person:

4 thin slices of sliced cheese (Gouda, Emmentaler or Tilsiter) | 1 tbsp cream cheese | 1/2 teaspoon of parsley chopped | 1 tbsp milk | 2 slices of poultry ham

Preparation:

1.   Dice the ham very finely and stir well with the cream cheese, parsley, and milk.

2.   Brush the cheese with this mass and roll it up.

3.   You can enjoy the rolls purely for breakfast or as a snack.

4.   You can also cut the rolls into rings and refine a small green salad.

5.   This makes for a great, light lunch - not just for hot summer days.

6.   Marinate the salad discreetly with some apple cider vinegar and oil.

Calories: 86.5 kcal | Protein: 10.5 grams | Fat: 4.5 grams | Carbohydrates: 1 gram

Ingredients for one person:

2 egg whites | 20 ml of mineral water | 1 tablespoon of Bacon finely diced | 1/2 teaspoon of parsley chopped | some marjoram fresh | pepper from the grinder

Preparation:

1.	Whisk the egg whites well with the soda water.
2.	Fry the bacon crisply in a non-fat coated pan.
3.	Pour the egg over it and sprinkle with parsley, marjoram, and pepper from the mill.
4.	Fry for 2 minutes on each side.
5.	You do not need salt for this omelet, as the bacon is usually salty enough.
6.	If you want to make the omelet with a whole egg, you use a whole egg instead of 2 egg whites.

Calories: 300.2 kcal | Protein: 11 grams | Fat: 24.2 grams | Carbohydrates: 9.6 grams

Ingredients for one person:

150 grams of yogurt | 1 splash of sweetener | some abrasion of a Bio Orange untreated | 1 tsp of walnuts chopped | 1 tsp almonds chopped | 1 teaspoon of pecans chopped | 1/2 pinch of Himalayan salt

Preparation:

1.	Roast the chopped nuts dark in a non-fat, coated pan and allow to cool.
2.	The yogurt with the sweetener and the abrasion of the orange smoothly stir and discreetly season with a little Himalayan salt.
3.	Stir in the nuts.
4.	You can also taste this yogurt with cinnamon, clove powder or ginger powder to your heart's content.

Recipes For Ketogenic Lunches And Dinner

Calories: 225.1 kcal | Protein: 24.3 grams | Fat: 13.9 grams | Carbohydrates: 0.7 grams

Ingredients for one person:

100 grams beef tenderloin | 1 shallot | 1 pinch of cayenne pepper | 1 knife tip mustard sharp | 1 tsp chervil chopped | 1 egg yolk | 1 pinch of Himalayan salt | 1 dash of lemon juice
Preparation:
1.   Cut the meat into very small cubes, using a very sharp knife.
2.   Finely chop the shallot and mix it with the meat.
3.   Season with Cayenne pepper, mustard, chervil, Himalayan salt, and lemon juice.
4.   Stir in the egg yolks and serve well chilled.
5.   If you do not want to eat raw tartare, you can fry it for a minute from both sides.
6.   If your daily turnover allows, you can also enjoy a slice of protein bread to Tartar.

Calories: 219 kcal | Protein: 32.5 grams | Fat: 8.6 grams | Carbohydrates: 2.9 grams
Ingredients for one person:
250 ml vegetable broth | 80 grams of chicken fillet | 1/2 bar of celery 20 grams of cauliflower | Salt and pepper | 1 laurel leaf | 1 egg | 1 tbsp chives cut in rolls
Preparation:
1.   Season the broth with salt, pepper and bring to the boil with the bay leaf.
2.   Cut the meat into 1.5 cm cubes and add to the hot soup.
3.   Simmer over medium heat for about 9 minutes.
4.   Cut the celery and cauliflower into bite-sized pieces and cook for 3 minutes.
5.   Just before the end, beat the egg into the boiling soup and stir with the whisk.
6.   Serve and sprinkle generously with chives.

Calories: 390.9 kcal | Protein: 34.2 grams | Fat: 26.9 grams | Carbohydrates: 3 grams
Ingredients for one person:
For the Hack-Balls:

140 grams of ground beef lean | 1 tablespoon coriander chopped | some abrasion of a bio lime | Salt and pepper | 1 egg yolk

For the sauce:

1/2 red onion | 1 clove of garlic | 1 teaspoon butter | 1/2 teaspoon yellow, Indian curry powder | Juice of half an organic lime | 80 ml of broth | 1 pinch of cardamom ground | 1 small pinch of cinnamon | 2 tablespoons yogurt | some soy sauce light without added sugar | Oyster sauce without added sugar

Preparation:

1.   Knead the ground beef with the chopped coriander, grated lime, egg yolk, salt, and pepper.

2.   Shape into balls with wet hands and place on a baking sheet lined with baking paper.

3.   Heat the oven to 200 ° C and bake the balls for 10 minutes with top, bottom and bottom heat.

4.   You can also prepare these comfortably in Airfryer.

5.   For the sauce, finely chop the onion and garlic and place the butter. Sweat the butter lightly.

6.   Stir in the curry powder and fry briefly. Deglaze with the lime juice and pour in the broth.

7.   Slightly reduce the liquid and remove from heat.

8.   Stir in the yogurt with the whisk and season with cardamom and cinnamon.

9.   Season with soy sauce and oyster sauce, let the balls simmer briefly in the sauce, and serve.

Calories: 205.1 kcal | Protein: 28.4 grams | Fat: 9.1 grams | Carbohydrates: 2.4 grams

Ingredients for one person:

300 ml of broth | 2 laurel leaves | 1/2 tsp. Mustard seeds | 2 sprigs of thyme | 150 grams of Alaska Pollock | 1 shallot | 1/2 teaspoon butter | Juice of half a lemon | 1 tsp dill chopped | 20 ml of cream | salt and pepper

Preparation:

1.   Boil the broth with the bay leaves, mustard seeds, thyme and salt, and pepper.
2.   Cut the fish fillet into two equal pieces and cool the broth to 70 ° C.
3.   Poach the fish in it for about 12 minutes.
4.   In the meantime, cut the shallot into small pieces and sauté lightly in the butter.
5.   Deglaze with the juice of the lemon, stir in the dill and infuse with a creator of poaching water.
6.   Refine with the cream, season with salt and pepper, let reduce for a short time and arrange the sauce together with the Alaskan salmon.

Calories: 215.9 kcal | Protein: 36.7 grams | Fat: 6.7 grams | Carbohydrates: 2.2 grams
Ingredients for one person:
150 grams turkey steak | Salt and pepper | 1 tsp blue cheese (Gorgonzola or Bavaria Blue) | 1 tsp cream cheese | 1 knife tip mustard sharp | Chopped 1/2 teaspoon parsley
Preparation:
1.   Salt and pepper the meat on both sides.
2.   In a grill pan without fat, sauté for 90 seconds on each side.
3.   Remove from the pan and place it on the grill.
4.   Smooth the blue cheese with the cream cheese and mix with mustard and parsley.
5.   Spread on the meat and heat the oven to 180 ° Celsius.
6.   Cook the turkey steak with the top, bottom and bottom heat for 8 minutes, remove from the oven and simmer.

Calories: 374.1 kcal | Protein: 34 grams | Fat: 23.7 grams | Carbohydrates: 6.2 grams
Ingredients for one person:

100 grams beef tenderloin | 60 grams of mozzarella | 1 tbsp olive oil | 1 tbsp balsamic vinegar | some abrasion of an untreated organic lime | 10 grams of arugula salad | 1 tablespoon of pine nuts chopped and roasted | salt and pepper

Preparation:

1.   Place the meat between two pouches and tap very thinly with a plating machine.

2.   Put on a plate and grate the mozzarella and spread over it.

3.   Cover with rocket and sprinkle with the lime rub.

4.   Marinate with vinegar and oil, salt and pepper and sprinkle generously with the pine nuts.

Calories: 362.3 kcal | Protein: 32.9 grams | Fat: 23.1 grams | Carbohydrates: 5.7 grams

Ingredients for one person:

150 grams of pikeperch skin without skin | Salt and pepper | 1 clove of garlic | sóme lemon juice | 15 grams of sesame white | 15 grams of sesame black | 1 tbsp sesame oil

Preparation:

1.   Chop the garlic very finely, salt the fish fillet and pepper and rub with the garlic.

2.   Drizzle with the lemon juice.

3.   Mix the sesame seeds and roll the fish in it.

4.   Press the sesame well.

5.   Roast the fish in hot sesame oil for 90 seconds on each side, remove from the pan and enjoy.

Calories: 167.5 kcal | Protein: 13.5 grams | Fat: 10.3 grams | Carbohydrates: 5.2 grams

Ingredients for one person:

60 grams of konjac noodles | 1/4 red onion | 1 clove of garlic | 60 grams of ground beef lean | 1 tbsp olive oil | 80 grams of canned pizza without added sugar | Salt and pepper | 1/2 teaspoon dried oregano | Fresh basil | 1 pinch of caraway ground | 1 dash of sweetener

Preparation:

1.	Finely chop the onion and garlic and fry in the olive oil.
2.	Add the meat and fry.
3.	Add the pizza tomato and season with salt, pepper, and oregano.
4.	Season with cumin and sweetener and simmer for 15 minutes.
5.	Rinse the Konjag noodles according to the package instructions and prepare, mix with the sauce and serve.
6.	Garnish with fresh basil before serving.
7.	If you want, you can refine the noodles with a teaspoon of freshly grated Parmesan.

Calories: 189.6 kcal | Protein: 21.2 grams | Fat: 10.8 grams | Carbohydrates: 1.9 grams

Ingredients for one person:

120 grams of squid | Salt and pepper | 1 tbsp cream cheese | 1 egg yolk | 1 tablespoon of parsley chopped | 1 chili red chopped | 1/2 teaspoon dill chopped | 1/4 red paprika finely diced

Preparation:

1.	Wash the squid and salt and pepper outside and inside.
2.	Smooth the cream cheese with the egg yolks and mix with the chopped parsley, chili, dill and paprika cubes.
3.	Fill the octopus with it and place it on a baking sheet lined with baking paper.
4.	Heat the oven to 190 ° Celsius and bake the octopus on top and bottom. Heat for 8 minutes.
5.	You can also prepare the squid comfortably in the Airfryer's Garkorb.

6.   If necessary, you can sprinkle the squid with a little fresh lemon juice.

Calories: 255.2 kcal | Protein: 28.8 grams | Fat: 14.8 grams | Carbohydrates: 1.7 grams
Ingredients for one person:
130 grams of chicken hearts | 1 shallot | 2 garlic cloves | 1 tbsp butter 50 ml of broth | some thyme | salt and pepper
Preparation:
1.   Finely chop the shallot and garlic and halve the chicken hearts.
2.   Fry them together with shallot and garlic in butter for 4 minutes.
3.   Add the stock and simmer for 3 minutes over medium heat.
4.   Season with thyme and season with salt and pepper as needed.
5.   If you want, you can refine this dish with a teaspoon of sour cream.

Calories: 71 kcal | Protein: 13.1 grams | Fat: 1 gram | Carbohydrates: 2.4 grams
Ingredients for one person:
1/2 tsp curry paste red | 200 ml vegetable broth | 2 lime leaves | 1/2 cm ginger | 4 shrimps without peel and cleaned | 2 cherry tomatoes | 2 mushrooms | Soy sauce light with no added sugar | Fish sauce without added sugar | 1 dash of sweetener
Preparation:
1.   Roast the curry paste in the wok without oil for about 3 minutes and pour in the vegetable broth.
2.   Stir well with the whisk until the paste has completely dissolved.
3.   Add the lime leaves and ginger and cook briefly.
4.   Quarter the shrimp and add to the soup. Cook for 4 minutes.

5.   Halve the tomatoes and mushrooms and add to the soup.

6.   Cook for another 3 minutes.

7.   Season with soy sauce, fish sauce, and sweetener.

8.   If necessary, you can sprinkle the soup with fresh, chopped cilantro.

Calories: 163.6 kcal | Protein: 26.9 grams | Fat: 5.6 grams | Carbohydrates: 1.4 grams

Ingredients for one person:

130 grams salmon fillet without skin | Salt and pepper | some lemon juice | 1 pinch of ginger freshly grated | 1/2 tsp tarragon chopped | 1 tbsp sour cream | 1 knife tip wasabi | 1 tablespoon of water | 1 tablespoon of apple cider vinegar | 10 grams of baby leaf spinach

Preparation:

1.   Finely dice the salmon with a sharp knife.

2.   Mix with salt, pepper, lemon juice, ginger, and tarragon and serve as tartar on a plate.

3.   Spread the spinach on the tartar.

4.   From the sour cream, the wasabi, the water, and the apple cider vinegar stir dressing and discreetly season with salt and pepper.

5.   Distribute over the leaf spinach, serve and enjoy.

6.   If you do not want to eat the tartare raw, you can mix an egg white under the salmon and cook it for 2 minutes on each side in a non-oiled frying pan.

Calories: 232 kcal | Protein: 37.8 grams | Fat: 14.8 grams | Carbohydrates: 5.4 grams

Ingredients for one person:

160 grams of turkey breast | 1/2 onion | 2 garlic cloves | 1 tablespoon vegetable oil | 1/2 teaspoon tomato paste without added sugar | 1/2 teaspoon paprika smoked mild | 1 pinch of paprika powder sharp | 2 tablespoons of apple cider vinegar | 200 ml vegetable broth | some marjoram dried | 1 pinch of caraway ground | 1 pinch of ginger finely grated | Salt and pepper | 2 tbsp sour cream
Preparation:
1.   Cut the turkey breast into 2 cm cubes, roughly chop the onion and garlic and fry until golden brown in the vegetable oil for about 5 minutes.
2.   Add the tomato paste and roast briefly.
3.   Cook the paprika mild and spicy for another minute.
4.   Add the apple cider vinegar and add the broth.
5.   Add the marjoram, cumin, and ginger and simmer the goulash for about 20 minutes over medium heat.
6.   Stir in a spoonful of sour cream and season to taste with salt and pepper.
7.   Arrange the goulash and garnish with the second spoon of sour cream.

Calories: 277.5 kcal | Protein: 29.1 grams | Fat: 16.7 grams | Carbohydrates: 2.7 grams
Ingredients for one person:
150 grams of venison | Salt and pepper | 1 sprig of thyme | 1 garlic clove with shell | 1 tbsp butter 1 shallot | 1 tablespoon diced bacon | 20 grams of boletus | 20 grams of chanterelles | 1 tablespoon of apple cider vinegar | 50 ml broth or stock | 1 tbsp sour cream | 1 tablespoon of parsley chopped
Preparation:
1.   Divide the venison into three equally sized medallions and salt and pepper on both sides.
2.   Sauté with the thyme and garlic in the butter all around for about 3 minutes.
3.   Remove the meat from the pan and place it on a grill.

4.	Cover with thyme and garlic and cook at 100 ° C for 10 minutes at the top and bottom. Heat.
5.	So you get the cooking level pink.
6.	In the meantime, cut the shallot into small pieces and roast golden-brown together with the bacon in the pan that has just been used.
7.	Cut the mushrooms into small pieces and add. Fry for about 2 minutes and deglaze with the apple cider vinegar.
8.	Add the broth and simmer for about 3 minutes.
9.	Season with salt and pepper and refine with the sour cream.
10. Serve the meat with the mushroom sauce.
Recipes For Ketogenic Snacks

Calories: 174.2 kcal | Protein: 13.7 grams | Fat: 12.2 grams | Carbohydrates: 2.4 grams
Ingredients for one person:
2 hard-boiled eggs | 1 tbsp. Creme Fraiche | 1/4 bar of celery 10 grams of cucumber | 1/2 tsp mustard sharp | Salt and pepper | 1 tablespoon of apple cider vinegar | 1 spring onion
Preparation:
1.	Cut the celery and cucumber into small pieces, chop the egg roughly and mix carefully.
2.	From the cream Fraiche, the mustard, salt, pepper and apple cider vinegar stir a creamy dressing and marinate the salad with it.
3.	Serve and sprinkle generously with the finely chopped spring onion.

Calories: 40.9 kcal | Protein: 4.6 grams | Fat: 0.5 grams | Carbohydrates: 4.5 grams
Ingredients for one person:
2 bars of celery 1 tbsp cream cheese | 1 tbsp. Curd | 1 splash of lemon juice | 1 clove of garlic | 1 tsp parsley roughly chopped | salt and pepper
Preparation:

1.	Peel the celery and cut into 5 cm pieces.
2.	Smooth the cream cheese with the quark and mix with lemon juice and finely chopped garlic.
3.	Season with salt and pepper and stir in the parsley.
4.	Enjoy the dip together with the celery.

Calories: 126.9 kcal | Protein: 12.3 grams | Fat: 5.3 grams | Carbohydrates: 7.5 grams
Ingredients for one person:
150 grams of yogurt | 2 egg whites | Juice of a lemon | 1/2 cm ginger fresh | Sweetener as needed
Preparation:
1.	Finely grate the ginger and stir together with the yogurt and the lemon juice.
2.	Beat the egg whites into a stiff snow and fold gently.
3.	Season with sweetener as needed and enjoy.
4.	This protein booster is also ideal as a small midnight snack, as it excites the metabolism during sleep excellently.

Calories: 111.7 kcal | Protein: 9.9 grams | Fat: 7.3 grams | Carbohydrates: 1.6 grams
Ingredients for one person:
1 egg | 30 ml of milk | Salt and pepper | 1 pinch of nutmeg grated | 1/2 teaspoon of parsley chopped | 1 tablespoon of gouda grated
Preparation:
1.	Whisk the egg with the milk, season with salt, pepper and nutmeg and flavor with the parsley.
2.	Pour into a small casserole dish and sprinkle with the Gouda.
3.	Stir in the oven at 170 ° C and circulating air for 10 minutes.

Calories: 250.2 kcal | Protein: 22.2 grams | Fat: 17.4 grams | Carbohydrates: 1.2 grams
Ingredients for one person:

60 grams of parmesan finely grated | 1 teaspoon rosemary finely chopped | 1 pinch of paprika powder

Preparation:

1.   Mix the parmesan with the rosemary and the paprika powder well.

2.   Layout a baking tray with parchment paper and place small heaps of cheese on it with a spoon.

3.   Pay attention to sufficient distance.

4.   Heat the oven to 200 ° Celsius and bake the chips for 4 minutes with top, bottom and bottom heat.

5.   Remove from the oven, let cool and use it as a great alternative to potato chips and coals snack.

Calories: 361.7 kcal | Protein: 25.8 grams | Fat: 27.8 grams | Carbohydrates: 2.3 grams

Ingredients for one person:

1 camembert 125 grams | 1/2 pepper green | 1 tbsp chives in rolls

Preparation:

1.   Cut the camembert on the surface with a cross.

2.   Place on a tray lined with baking paper and preheat the oven to 180 ° Celsius.

3.   Heat the cheese in circulating air for about 8 minutes.

4.   Remove from the oven, sprinkle with chives, cut the peppers into strips and use for dipping.

Calories: 13.4 kcal | Protein: 1.3 grams | Fat: 0.2 grams | Carbohydrates: 1.6 grams

Ingredients for one person:

60 grams of pointed cabbage | Salt and pepper | some paprika powder

Preparation:

1.   Lay out a baking sheet with parchment paper and distribute the individual cabbage leaves on it.

2.   Season with salt, pepper, and paprika and heat the oven to 160 ° Celsius.

3.   Allow the cabbage to dry for 20 minutes at the top, bottom and bottom heat to crisps.

Calories: 177.5 kcal | Protein: 14.1 grams | Fat: 11.9 grams | Carbohydrates: 3.5 grams
Ingredients for one person:
1/2 ball mozzarella | 1 small tomato | 1 tbsp balsamic vinegar | 1 tbsp extra virgin olive oil | 6 sheets of basil | 1/2 onion red | 1 pinch of sea salt | colorful pepper from the mill
Preparation:
1.   Pick the mozzarella into bite-sized pieces, dice the tomato and marinate with vinegar and oil.
2.   Chop the basil roughly and cut the onions into strips.
3.   Also, fold in, arrange and sprinkle with sea salt and colorful, freshly ground pepper.

Calories: 99.7 kcal | Protein: 6.8 grams | Fat: 5.3 grams | Carbohydrates: 6.2 grams
Ingredients for one person:
150 grams of yogurt | 1 splash of lime juice | 1 pinch of cinnamon | 1 pinch of turmeric | 1 pinch of cardamom ground | 1 pinch of clove powder | 1 pinch of ginger powder | 1 pinch of cayenne pepper | Sweetener as needed
Preparation:
1.   Mix the lime juice with the yogurt until smooth and stir in all the spices with the whisk.
2.   Let the spices soak for a few minutes, sweeten with sweetener as needed and enjoy.

Calories: 104 kcal | Protein: 12.7 grams | Fat: 4.4 grams | Carbohydrates: 3.4 grams
Ingredients for one person:
100 grams of cottage cheese grainy | 1 splash of sweetener | 1 knife tip double de-oiled cocoa powder | 1 pinch of cinnamon | 2 tablespoons cold coffee
Preparation:

1.   Mix the cottage cheese with the cold coffee and the sweetener and season with cocoa and cinnamon.
2.   Let it through briefly and enjoy.
3.   Of course, you can also spice up the cottage cheese with cayenne pepper, a pinch of salt and fresh herbs.

Recipes For Ketogenic Drinks

Calories: 14.1 kcal | Protein: 0.4 grams | Fat: 0.1 grams | Carbohydrates: 2.9 grams
Ingredients for one person:
1/4 cucumber | 1/2 cm ginger fresh | 1/2 bunch of coriander | Juice of half a lime | 150 ml of cold tea of your choice - the best are herbal teas or green tea | Sweetener as needed
Preparation:
1.   Add all ingredients to the Blender or Smoothie Maker and add to a creamy drink.
2.   Sweeten and enjoy as needed.
3.   On hot days, you can, of course, serve the drink with a few ice cubes, which you can also add to the blender.

Calories: 33 kcal | Protein: 2.2 grams | Fat: 1.8 grams | Carbohydrates: 2 grams
Ingredients for one person:
150 ml of green tea | 1 pinch of vanilla or a few drops of vanilla flavor 1 splash of sweetener | 50 grams of yogurt
Preparation:
1.   Mix all ingredients in a blender or with a whisk.
2.   Enjoy hot or cold.

Calories: 64.1 kcal | Protein: 8.4 grams | Fat: 0.9 grams | Carbohydrates: 5.6 grams
Ingredients for one person:
150 ml of milk | 1 tbsp cream cheese | 20 grams of Whey powder with chocolate flavor | 1/2 tsp double de-oiled cocoa | some sweetener | 1 pinch of Himalayan salt
Preparation:

1.	Add all ingredients to the blender or smoothie maker and stir well.
2.	You can also make the Keto Chocolate Shake hot.
3.	To make the Bullet Proof cocoa, add a spoonful of butter.
4.	A spoonful of butter in your daily coffee will also help you with the ketogenic diet.

Calories: 2.6 kcal | Protein: 0.2 grams | Fat: 0.2 grams | Carbohydrates: 0 grams
Ingredients for one person:
150 ml Cola light | some rum aroma | 1/2 lime | 1 glass with ice cube
Preparation:
1.	Cut the lime into thin slices and add it to the ice cubes.
2.	Fill up the Diet Coke and drizzle with Rum Aroma.
3.	Serve with a straw - so you survive any party without giving up your keto diet.

Calories: 162.3 kcal | Protein: 1.2 grams | Fat: 13.1 grams | Carbohydrates: 9.9 grams
Ingredients for one person:
100 ml of coconut milk | 50 grams of fresh pineapple | Juice of a lime | 1/2 glass of ice cubes
Preparation:
1.	Pour the coconut milk with the pineapple and the lime juice into the blender or smoothie maker and then pour over the ice cubes.
2.	This alcohol-free cocktail is sure to be the absolute star at every garden party.

Calories: 10 kcal | Protein: 1.3 grams | Fat: 0.4 grams | Carbohydrates: 0.3 grams
Ingredients for one person:
200 ml of green tea | 1 tsp matcha powder | 1 tbsp cottage cheese | 1 splash of sweetener | 1 pinch of sea salt

Preparation:

1.   Mix all ingredients in the blender or smoothie maker to a creamy shake.

2.   Matcha is not only good for the immune system, the special green tea is rich in vitamins and minerals and boosts the metabolism really.

Calories: 36.5 kcal | Protein: 0.8 grams | Fat: 1.7 grams | Carbohydrates: 4.5 grams

Ingredients for one person:

150 ml almond milk | 15 grams of moring leaves fresh or powder | 1 pinch of cardamom ground | 1 small pinch of Himalayan salt | Sweetener as needed

Preparation:

1.   Mix all the ingredients in the blender or smoothie maker to a creamy shake.

2.   Sweeten and enjoy as needed.

3.   Moringa is considered an absolute superfood and is known as a scavenger of free radicals as a true fountain of youth.

Calories: 0 kcal | Protein: 0 grams | Fat: 0 grams | Carbohydrates: 0 grams

Ingredients for one person:

1 liter of water | 5 cm ginger fresh | 1 red chili | 2 limes sliced

Preparation:

1.   Cut the ginger and chili into small pieces and place them together with the lime slices in a jug of water.

2.   You can refill the pitcher with water and drink the detox water all day long.

3.   To cleanse the intestines you can mix a glass of water with a spoon of Glauber's salt in the morning or in the evening.

Recipes For Ketogenic Desserts

Calories: 328 kcal | Protein: 6.9 grams | Fat: 30 grams | Carbohydrates: 7.6 grams

Ingredients for one person:

150 ml of cream | 2 sheets of gelatine | Mark of a half vanilla pod | Sweetener as needed

Preparation:

1.   Boil the cream with the vanilla once and sweeten as needed.
2.   Allow to cool slightly.
3.   Soak the gelatine in water, squeeze it out and dissolve quickly in the still-warm cream.
4.   Stir well with the whisk to avoid lumps.
5.   Pour into a pudding tin and chill for about 6 hours.

Calories: 157.4 kcal | Protein: 8 grams | Fat: 11 grams | Carbohydrates: 6.6 grams

Ingredients for one person:

100 ml of buttermilk | 2 sheets of gelatine | 50 ml of cream | Sweetener as needed | 2 drops of mint flavor

Preparation:

1.   Lightly warm the buttermilk and sweeten as needed.
2.   Soak the gelatine in water, squeeze and dissolve in the warm buttermilk.
3.   Stir well with the whisk to avoid lumps.
4.   Beat the cream with the mint aroma until stiff and place it under the buttermilk.
5.   Put in a bowl and refrigerate for about 4 hours.
6.   Of course, you can also use vanilla, chocolate or rum flavor.

Calories: 101.6 kcal | Protein: 15.8 grams | Fat: 1.6 grams | Carbohydrates: 6 grams

Ingredients for one person:

15 grams Low Carb Fitness Bar | 50 grams of cottage cheese with 0.5% FiT | some sweetener as needed | Juice and abrasion of a half untreated organic lime | 30 grams of raspberries fresh or frozen

Preparation:

1.   Crumble the Low Carb Fitness bar in a freezer bag and pour it into a glass.
2.   Smooth the quark with the sweetener, the rubbing and the juice of the lime and also layer it in the glass.
3.   Cover with the raspberries, let them soak in the fridge and enjoy.

Calories: 18.8 kcal | Protein: 4.3 grams | Fat: 0 grams | Carbohydrates: 0.4 grams

Ingredients for one person:

100 ml apple tea | a little vanilla aroma | 1 splash of lime juice | 1 splash of sweetener | 3 sheets of gelatine

Preparation:

1.   Boil the apple tea with the vanilla flavor, the lime juice, and the sweetener briefly and allow it to cool.
2.   Soak the gelatine in water, squeeze well and dissolve in the still-warm tea.
3.   Fill the liquid in a small bowl and leave it in the fridge for at least 3 hours.

Calories: 14.4 kcal | Protein: 3.3 grams | Fat: 0 grams | Carbohydrates: 0.3 grams

Ingredients for one person:

1 egg white | 20 ml of soda water | some sweetener | some abrasion of an untreated organic lemon

Preparation:

1.   Beat the egg whites with soda and process to a stiff snow.
2.   Then gently fold in the sweetener and the lemons.
3.   Form small cams on a baking sheet lined with baking paper and heat the oven to 130 ° Celsius.

4.   Allow the meringue to dry for 25 minutes in the top and bottom heat.

Calories: 180.1 kcal | Protein: 10.3 grams | Fat: 14.5 grams | Carbohydrates: 2.1 grams

Ingredients for one person:

1 egg | 2 tablespoons milk | 1 tbsp almond flour | 1 tbsp. Curd | 1/2 tsp double de-oiled cocoa | some sweetener | 1/2 teaspoon butter

Preparation:

1.   Whisk the egg with the milk and stir in the almond flour.

2.   Bake in a pan in hot butter to an omelet.

3.   Smooth the quark with the cocoa and sweetener and fill with the omelet.

4.   Sprinkle with powdered xylitol as needed.

5.   You can also enjoy the omelet with a small amount of cream.

Calories: 154.2 kcal | Protein: 9.1 grams | Fat: 11.4 grams | Carbohydrates: 3.8 grams

Ingredients for one person:

1 egg | 1 tbsp almonds grated | 50 grams berry mix fresh or TK | Powder xylitol or sweetener as needed

Preparation:

1.   Separate the egg and process the egg white into a stiff snow.

2.   Mix the egg yolks with the grated almonds and season with a little sweetener.

3.   Add the egg whites and put the berries in a casserole dish.

4.   Cover the berries with the egg mass.

5.   Preheat the oven to 190 ° C and bake the gratin for 7 minutes in the top and bottom heat.

6.   Sprinkle with powdered xylitol as needed.

Chapter 8 - Plan For Your Ketogenic Diet

This plan consists of a suggestion for lunch and dinner. You can, of course, change your meals individually, but always keep an eye on your total carbohydrate intake.

Day 1:
Calories: 213.7 kcal | Protein: 14.4 grams | Fat: 16.1 grams | Carbohydrates: 2.8 grams
Ingredients for one person:
1 shallot | 1 clove of garlic | 1/2 teaspoon butter | 30 grams of leaf spinach | 2 eggs | Salt and pepper | 1 tbsp ricotta
Preparation:
1.	Cut the shallot and garlic into small pieces and fry in a glassy sauce.
2.	Add the leaf spinach and lightly collapse in the heat.
3.	Put the vegetables in a small baking dish.
4.	Then spread the ricotta.
5.	Whisk the eggs with salt and pepper and pour over the leaf spinach.
6.	Heat the oven to 200 ° Celsius and bake the frittata for 10 minutes with top, bottom and bottom heat.
Calories: 314.1 kcal | Protein: 41.4 grams | Fat: 15.3 grams | Carbohydrates: 2.7 grams
Ingredients for one person:
150 grams of turkey breast | Salt and pepper | 1 tbsp butter 1 egg | 1 tbsp chives in rolls | 2 small gherkins without added sugar
Preparation:
1.	Tap the turkey breast thinly, salt and pepper and fry in butter from both sides for 2 minutes until golden brown.
2.	Fry the fried eggs next to the meat in the same pan.
3.	Arrange the meat, put the fried egg on top, sprinkle with the chives and decorate with the gürkchen.
Day 2:

Calories: 347.6 kcal | Protein: 23.5 grams | Fat: 26.8 grams | Carbohydrates: 3.1 grams

Ingredients for one person:

100 grams Halloumi barbecue cheese | 2 slices of turkey ham | 3 cherry tomatoes | 1 sprig of rosemary | salt and pepper

Preparation:

1.   Grill the cheese in a non-fat frying pan for 2 minutes on each side.

2.   Skew the tomatoes on the rosemary branch and fry in the pan.

3.   Season with salt and pepper and arrange the cheese with the ham and tomatoes.

4.   You can leave the ham raw, or you can also fry it briefly in the pan.

Calories: 168.8 kcal | Protein: 21.7 grams | Fat: 8.4 grams | Carbohydrates: 1.6 grams

Ingredients for one person:

140 grams of prawns without shell and cleaned | 2 garlic cloves | 1 tbsp butter | Juice and abrasion of a half untreated organic lemon | 2 tablespoons of zucchini diced | Salt and pepper | 1 tablespoon parsley roughly chopped

Preparation:

1.   Cut the garlic leafy and discard with the shrimp in butter for 3 minutes.

2.   Flavor with the juice and abrasion of the lemon.

3.   Add the diced zucchini, lightly salt and pepper and fry for another 2 minutes.

4.   Before serving, sprinkle generously with parsley.

Day 3:

Calories: 183.4 kcal | Protein: 21.5 grams | Fat: 10.2 grams | Carbohydrates: 1.4 grams

Ingredients for one person:

1 shallot | 1 teaspoon butter | 100 grams salmon fillet without skin | 2 eggs | 1 tbsp cream cheese | 1 tablespoon chopped chili | Salt and pepper | 3 tomato slices for garnish

Preparation:

1.   Cut the shallot into small pieces and fry in a glassy sauce.

2.   Cut the salmon into 1 cm cubes and add to the pan.

3.   Whisk the eggs with the cream cheese and season with chervil, salt, and pepper.

4.   Pour over the fish and cook over medium heat while stirring constantly.

5.   Serve and garnish with the tomatoes, sprinkle with fresh herbs as needed.

Calories: 249.2 kcal | Protein: 29,6 grams | Fat: 12.8 grams | Carbohydrates: 3.9 grams

Ingredients for one person:

150 grams beef tenderloin | Salt and steak pepper | 1 red onion | 1 tbsp butter | 2 tablespoons of apple cider vinegar | 1 splash of sweetener | some thyme

Preparation:

1.   Season the beef filet with salt and steak pepper and sauté in a grill pan from both sides for 2 minutes each.

2.   Place on the grill and finish cooking at 100 ° C for 15 minutes.

3.   Slice the onion and fry in butter until translucent.

4.   After 4 minutes deglaze with the apple cider vinegar and season with sweetener.

5.   Aroma with thyme and serve with the steak.

Day 4:

Calories: 474,6 kcal | Protein: 32 grams | Fat: 36.2 grams | Carbohydrates: 5.2 grams

Ingredients for one person:

4 slices of bacon | 1 pinch of cinnamon | 1/2 teaspoon maple syrup | 2 eggs | 1 Early Ling onion

Preparation:

1.   Season the bacon with cinnamon and maple syrup in a non-stick pan, fry crispy on both sides.

2.   Push the bacon to the edge of the pan and roast the fried eggs in the spilled oil.

3.   Arrange this with the crispy bacon and serve generously with finely chopped spring onion.

Calories: 269.5 kcal | Protein: 29.7 grams | Fat: 15.1 grams | Carbohydrates: 3.7 grams

Ingredients for one person:

150 grams of fillet of ostrich | 1 tbsp olive oil | Salt and pepper | 1 shallot | 1 pinch of tomato paste without added sugar | 1 pinch of paprika powder sharp | 1/4 bell pepper yellow | 1/4 red bell pepper | 50 ml vegetable broth | some marjoram dried | 1 tbsp sour cream | Parsley chopped to sprinkle

Preparation:

1.   Salt and pepper the meat and fry in olive oil for 2 minutes on each side.

2.   Remove from pan and keep in the oven at 80 ° C.

3.   Cut the shallot into small pieces and fry briefly in the same pan.

4.   Add the tomato paste and the paprika powder and roast briefly.

5.   Cut the peppers into thin strips and add to the pan.

6.   Swirl briefly and pour in the broth.

7.   Flavor with marjoram and put the meat in the pan.

8.   Cook at medium heat for 5 minutes.

9.   Season with salt and pepper, arrange and garnish with parsley and sour cream before serving.

Day 5:

Calories: 228.4 kcal | Protein: 31 grams | Fat: 11.2 grams | Carbohydrates: 0.9 grams

Ingredients for one person:

1 egg | 1 liter of vigorous vegetable broth | 50 ml of vinegar | 1 tablespoon salt | 100 grams of roast beef thinly sliced | 1 tbsp cottage cheese | 1 tsp chives in rolls | salt and pepper

Preparation:

1.   Bring the broth with the vinegar and salt to a boil and reduce the temperature to 70 ° C.

2.   Carefully poach the egg in it.

3.   Mix the cottage cheese with the chives, subtly salt and pepper and arrange the roast beef with the poached egg and the cottage cheese.

Calories: 136.8 kcal | Protein: 29 grams | Fat: 0.8 grams | Carbohydrates: 3.4 grams

Ingredients for one person:

150 grams of cottage cheese | 1 pinch of Himalayan salt | 1 pinch of cayenne pepper | 1/4 bell pepper yellow | 1 tomato | 1 tbsp sorrel chopped | 1/2 tsp tarragon chopped | 1 tsp coriander chopped

Preparation:

1.   Dice the peppers and tomatoes and mix them with the herbs.

2.   Stir under the quark and season with Himalayan salt and cayenne pepper.

3.   If it allows your daily total sales you can eat a slice of protein bread with this quark.

Day 6:

Calories: 340.8 kcal | Protein: 51.2 grams | Fat: 14.4 grams | Carbohydrates: 1.6 grams

Ingredients for one person:

150 grams of chicken breast | 1 slice of poultry ham | 1 tbsp cream cheese | 1 tbsp of pecan nuts chopped | 1 tsp. Mint chopped | salt and pepper

Preparation:

1.   Tap the chicken breast lightly, salt and pepper and cover with the ham.

2.   Mix the cream cheese with the chopped nuts and the mint and spread with the ham.

3.   Fold the meat and place it on a tray lined with baking paper.

4.   Heat the oven to 180 ° C and cook the meat for 15 minutes with top, bottom and bottom heat.

5.   The turkey tastes great with a small salad, which you can marinate with lemon juice and some yogurt.

Calories: 250.6 kcal | Protein: 52.4 grams | Fat: 2.6 grams | Carbohydrates: 4.4 grams

Ingredients for one person:

200 grams of cottage cheese | 1/2 lemon filleted | 20 grams of whey protein | 1 splash of sweetener | 1 pinch of Himalayan salt | 1 tbsp. Mint chocolate chopped

Preparation:

1.   Smooth the quark with the whey protein.

2.   Cut the lemon into small pieces and mix with the mint under the quark.

3.   Season with sweetener and rock salt and enjoy well chilled.

Day 7:

Calories: 233.4 kcal | Protein: 30.7 grams | Fat: 11.8 grams | Carbohydrates: 1.1 grams

Ingredients for one person:

140 grams of veal schnitzel | 1 tbsp cottage cheese | Salt and pepper | 2 radishes | 1/2 teaspoon sage finely chopped | 3 thin slices of black forest ham

Preparation:

1.   Tap the veal schnitzel thinly, salt and pepper.

2.   Grate the radishes finely and stir well with the cottage cheese and the sage.

3.   Spread the meat with it, make it into a roll and wrap it with the Black Forest ham.

4.   Sauté in a pan without oil.

5.   Place on a grill and cook in a 120 ° C oven for 10 minutes.

6.   Of course, you can also use chicken or turkey for this dish.

Calories: 360 kcal | Protein: 20.8 grams | Fat: 30 grams | Carbohydrates: 1.7 grams

Ingredients for one person:

2 eggs | 2 tablespoons yogurt | 1 pinch of yellow curry powder | some pepper white | 20 grams of blue cheese (Gorgonzola or Bavaria Blue) | 1 teaspoon butter | 1 teaspoon mountain cheese grated

Preparation:

1.	Stir the eggs with the yogurt, curry, and pepper until they are smooth.

2.	Stir in the hot butter.

3.	Spread the blue cheese over it, fold it up and sprinkle with the mountain cheese.

4.	Put the pan in the oven and cook for another 4 minutes with the grill function.

Day 8:

Calories: 357.3 kcal | Protein: 20.7 grams | Fat: 29.3 grams | Carbohydrates: 2.7 grams

Ingredients for one person:

10 grams of butter | 10 grams of almond flour | 50 ml of milk | Salt and pepper | 1 egg | 20 grams of parmesan finely grated | 2 thin slices of cooked ham

Preparation:

1.	Melt the butter in a small saucepan and quickly stir in the almond flour with the whisk.

2.	Add the milk and cook for 2 minutes, stirring constantly.

3.	Remove from the flame and allow it to cool slightly. Salt and pepper and separate the egg.

4.	The egg white to a stiff snow process.

5.	Stir the egg yolks and the Parmesan under the milk mixture.

6.	Cut the ham into small pieces and also add to it.

7.	Carefully fold in the egg whites and pour the mixture into a lightly buttered, refractory dish.

8.	Heat the oven to 200 ° Celsius and bake the souffle for 20 minutes in the top and bottom heat.

9.	Do not open the oven during baking.

Calories: 531.9 kcal | Protein: 36.4 grams | Fat: 40.3 grams | Carbohydrates: 5.9 grams

Ingredients for one person:

1 avocado | 80 grams of chicken breast | 1 shallot | 1 tsp olive oil | 1 tbsp walnuts chopped | 40 grams Camembert | salt and pepper

Preparation:

1.   Halve the avocado and free it from the core.
2.   With a spoon, gently scrape out the flesh and cut the flesh.
3.   Cut the chicken breast into thin strips, dice the shallot and sauté together in the olive oil for about 3 minutes.
4.   Add the nuts and the pulp, swirl briefly and fill in the avocado halves.
5.   Dice the camembert and spread on the avocado.
6.   Salt and pepper and place on a baking sheet lined with baking paper.
7.   Heat the oven to 200 ° Celsius and bake the avocado for 5 minutes at the top and bottom heat.

Day 9:

Calories: 280.6 kcal | Protein: 19.5 grams | Fat: 21 grams | Carbohydrates: 3.4 grams

Ingredients for one person:

6 bars of asparagus white | 6 thin slices of turkey ham | 1 egg | 1 tbsp almond flour | salt and pepper

Preparation:

1.   Peel the asparagus and free from the woody ends.
2.   Cook in salted water for about 10 minutes. Drain the water and quench the asparagus with cold water.
3.   Wrap the asparagus with the ham.
4.   Whisk the egg with the almond flour and season it discreetly with salt and pepper.
5.   Immerse the asparagus in the mass and place it on a baking sheet lined with baking paper.
6.   Heat the oven to 200 ° Celsius and bake the asparagus crispy for 5 minutes with top and bottom heat.

Calories: 377.2 kcal | Protein: 37.8 grams | Fat: 23.2 grams | Carbohydrates: 4.3 grams

Ingredients for one person:

150 grams lamb-back | 4 brown mushrooms | 2 garlic cloves | something rosemary | some thyme | Salt and pepper | 1 tbsp butter 1 teaspoon almond flour | 2 tablespoons sour cream | 1 tbsp. Mint finely chopped

Preparation:

1.   Cut the lamb into bite-sized cubes and thread them alternately with the mushrooms on a wooden skewer.

2.   Mince the garlic with the rosemary and thyme in a mortar.

3.   Rub the lamb with it, season with salt and pepper and fry in a pan in butter for one minute from each side.

4.   Place on a grill and cook for a further 12 minutes at 120 ° C and top, bottom and bottom heat.

5.   Now stir in the almond flour with the whisk into the pan you just used.

6.   Add the sour cream and let it rise with constant stirring.

7.   Stir in the mint, season with salt and pepper and arrange the sauce together with the skewer.

8.   If you do not like mint, you can, of course, use all herbs for the sauce.

Day 10:

Calories: 352.9 kcal | Protein: 48.5 grams | Fat: 16.5 grams | Carbohydrates: 2.6 grams

Ingredients for one person:

150 grams of tuna steak | Salt and pepper | some lemon juice | 1 egg | 2 tablespoons sour cream | 2 tablespoons almond flour | 1 tbsp carrot finely grated | 1/2 teaspoon dill chopped | 1/2 teaspoon butter

Preparation:

1.   Salt the tuna steak and pepper and drizzle with a little lemon juice.

2.   Fry for 2 minutes on each side in a grill pan without fat.

3.   Whisk the egg with the sour cream and stir with the almond flour.
4.   Add the grated carrot and the dill and season to taste with salt and pepper.
5.   Bake in a pan in hot butter to a pancake.
6.   Serve with the fish.
Calories: 97.9 kcal | Protein: 12.3 grams | Fat: 3.9 grams | Carbohydrates: 3.4 grams
Ingredients for one person:
200 ml of soy milk | 2 egg whites | 1 tbsp oat bran | 1 pinch of Himalayan salt | 1 dash of sweetener
Preparation:
1.   Add all ingredients to the Blender or the Smoothie Maker and process to a smooth shake.
2.   Best for 10 minutes in the fridge swell and then enjoy.
3.   This shake is also an ideal snack when cravings for sweets.

Day 11:

Calories: 398.5 kcal | Protein: 36.8 grams | Fat: 26.5 grams | Carbohydrates: 3.2 grams
Ingredients for one person:
100 grams of chicken breast | 1/2 onion red | 1 tsp olive oil | Salt and pepper | 1 small zucchini | 1/2 bunch of coriander | Roughly 1 tablespoon of walnuts | 2 tablespoons of walnut oil | Grated 1 tablespoon of parmesan
Preparation:
1.   Cut the chicken breast into thin strips and cut the onion into thin slices.
2.   Fry together in olive oil for 4 minutes.
3.   Salt and pepper and simmer on low heat.
4.   The zucchini with the peeler to & quot; noodles & quot; process and also put into the pan.
5.   Swirl for 4 minutes with the meat and the onion.
6.   In the meantime, add the coriander with the walnuts, walnut oil and Parmesan to the blender.
7.   To a creamy pesto process and lightly salt and pepper.

8.   Put the pesto in the pan, swing through and arrange.

9.   You can use any other nuts or seeds for the pesto.

10.   With pumpkin seeds, you get a very intense, aromatic pesto.

Calories: 419.1 kcal | Protein: 25.4 grams | Fat: 33.9 grams | Carbohydrates: 3.1 grams

Ingredients for one person:

60 grams of cooked ham | 1 shallot | 1 clove of garlic | 1 teaspoon butter | 2 eggs | 20 ml of cream | Salt and pepper | some marjoram dried | 1 tsp chives in rolls

Preparation:

1.   Cut the ham into thin strips and finely chop the shallot and garlic.

2.   Brown together in the butter until golden brown.

3.   Whisk the eggs with the cream, season with salt and pepper and flavor with marjoram.

4.   Pour over the ham and let it cook slowly over low heat.

5.   Rip with a wooden spoon to a scrambled egg, arrange and sprinkle generously with chives before serving.

Day 12:

Calories: 505.9 kcal | Protein: 62.6 grams | Fat: 25.9 grams | Carbohydrates: 5.6 grams

Ingredients for one person:

140 grams of poultry minced | 1 egg | 1/2 tsp. Mustard spicy with no added sugar | 1 red chili | 1/2 cm ginger fresh | 1/2 onion | 1 clove of garlic | 1/2 teaspoon butter | 30 grams of mountain cheese spicy | 1 tablespoon of parsley finely chopped | 1 tbsp oat bran | Salt and pepper | some dried thyme

Preparation:

1.   Mix the minced meat with the egg and mustard well.

2.   Chop chili, ginger, and garlic and sauté in butter for 2 to 3 minutes.

3.   Then add to the minced meat and pass through.

4.   Chop the mountain cheese into small pieces and add to the minced meat together with the parsley, oat bran and thyme.

5.   Salt and pepper and knead well.

6.   Mold loaves with wet hands and fry them in a nonstick pan in a nonstick pan.

7.   You should fry the patties on each side for about 3 minutes.

8.   If you want to eat ketchup with your loaf, you should make sure that you use ketchup without added sugar.

Calories: 297,6 kcal | Protein: 14.7 grams | Fat: 25.2 grams | Carbohydrates: 3 grams

Ingredients for one person:

2 eggs | 1 pinch of cinnamon | a little vanilla aroma | 2 tablespoon sour cream | 1 splash of sweetener | 1 tablespoon of hazelnuts finely chopped | 1/2 teaspoon butter | 1 pinch of Himalayan salt

Preparation:

1.   Whisk the eggs with the sour cream and stir until smooth with the cinnamon and vanilla flavor.

2.   Season with salt and sweetener.

3.   Lightly roast the hazelnuts in the butter and pour the egg over it.

4.   Stir for 3 minutes and tear with the wooden spoon to a nice scrambled egg.

Day 13:

Calories: 255 kcal | Protein: 11.2 grams | Fat: 21.8 grams | Carbohydrates: 3.5 grams

Ingredients for one person:

1 shallot | 1/2 teaspoon butter | 2 tablespoons of apple cider vinegar | 150 ml vegetable broth | 1 tbsp Rubbed Gouda | 1 tablespoon of Tilsiter grated | 50 ml of coconut milk | Salt and pepper | 1 pinch of anise powder | 1/2 teaspoon of Parmesan | 1/2 teaspoon grated coconut

Preparation:

1.   Finely chop the shallot and fry in a glassy sauce.

2.   Douse with the apple cider vinegar and let the liquid almost completely reduce.

3.   Add the broth and bring to a boil.

4.   Stir Gouda and Tilsiter and let it melt over medium heat with constant stirring.

5.   Stir in the coconut milk and season with salt, pepper, and anise.

6.   In the meantime roast the grated coconut in a pan without oil until dark.

7.   Arrange the soup, sprinkle with Parmesan and grated coconut and enjoy.

8.   You can, of course, use any cheese of your choice for this cheese soup.

Calories: 274,6 kcal | Protein: 22.4 grams | Fat: 17.8 grams | Carbohydrates: 6.2 grams

Ingredients for one person:

80 grams of mussels without shell | 1/4 onion red | 1 tbsp butter 1/2 bar of celery 2 eggs | 2 tablespoons sour cream | 10 grams of bean sprouts | 1 tsp chervil chopped | salt and pepper

Preparation:

1.   Dice the onion and cook with the mussels in the butter for about 2 minutes.

2.   Cut the celery into thin slices and add.

3.   Fry for another 3 minutes.

4.   Whisk the eggs with the sour cream and season with salt and pepper.

5.   Stir in the chervil and pour the egg over the mussels.

6.   Close the pan with a lid and let the omelet stand well for about 3 minutes with low heat.

7.   Remove the lid, spread the bean sprouts on the omelet, leave for a minute and arrange.

Day 14:

Calories: 378.1 kcal | Protein: 19.1 grams | Fat: 32.1 grams | Carbohydrates: 3.2 grams

Ingredients for one person:

1 shallot | 1 clove of garlic | 1 teaspoon butter | 60 grams of leaf spinach | 50 grams of sour cream | Salt and pepper | some nutmeg grated | Dried marjoram | 2 slices of ham | 1 egg | 1 pinch of paprika powder

Preparation:

1.   Chop the shallot and garlic and fry in butter until translucent.

2.   Coarsely chop the spinach and add.

3.   Let the spinach collapse, stir in the sour cream and season with salt, pepper, and nutmeg.

4.   Flavor with marjoram.

5.   Fry the ham crispy on both sides in a non-stick pan.

6.   Whisk the egg with salt, pepper, and paprika, pour on the ham and let it stand for 2 minutes.

7.   Then turn and fry for another minute. Serve and enjoy with the spinach.

Calories: 397,5 kcal | Protein: 53.1 grams | Fat: 19.9 grams | Carbohydrates: 1.5 grams

Ingredients for one person:

140 grams of chicken breast | Salt and pepper | 1 tbsp almond flour | 1 egg | 2 tablespoons cream | 1/2 teaspoon of parsley chopped | 1/2 tsp coriander chopped | some fresh thyme | 3 needles of rosemary finely chopped | 1 tbsp butter

Preparation:

1.   Tap the chicken breast very thinly, salt, pepper and toss in almond flour.

2.   Whisk the egg with the cream, salt and pepper, and flavor with parsley, coriander, thyme, and rosemary.

3.   Pull the chicken breast through the egg and sauté in the pan with hot butter.

4.   Pour over the rest of the egg and turn after about 3 minutes.

5.   Fry and serve for another 2 minutes.

Conclusion

Thank you for making it through to the end of *Ketogenic Diet: What It Is And How It Works*, let's hope it was informative and able to provide you with all of the tools you need to achieve your goals whatever they may be.

If you've been through the first few days of your diet, you can have a little cheat day. When doing this, you should not feast but be unrestrained. But you may, for example, enjoy a small portion of carbohydrates as a side dish for lunch. But maybe you also feel like spaghetti - but remember not to overdo it.

Once you have reached your desired weight, you should increase the enjoyment of carbohydrates slowly and not immediately fall back into old patterns. It is important to keep your weight in the long term is that you also in the future once a week a strict ketogenic day. So your weight can always swing out and the yo-yo effect cannot harm you.

We wish you a good success and hope that our recipes will taste good and accompany you on the way to the desired weight.

Finally, if you found this book useful in any way, a review on Amazon is always appreciated!

Description

In addition to the right diet, of course, the movement plays a major role. To get the metabolism going in the morning, you should schedule a small training session every day in the morning. It takes 10 minutes. You can dance, do sit-ups, get on the exercise bike or look for a variety of aerobics and workouts on YouTube. Here is the right thing for every taste and you'll see how energetic you start the day.

Equally important is to drink enough. Really try to consume 3 liters of water daily. You should resort to high-quality mineral water. Better is always still water. If water is too boring for you alone, you can flavor it with fresh herbs, ginger, cinnamon, cloves, and sliced citrus fruits.

Any diet is easier if you can do it with someone together. If you can not persuade your family to do so, maybe a friend would like it. So you can also exchange your successes daily and motivate each other. Also, a new hobby makes sure that you distract yourself and your thoughts do not have to constantly turn to food.

This book will teach you that it is very important that you always take the time to eat. You should never be distracted while doing so. So you outsmart your body, as it focuses on the food and gets full faster. The newspaper or the Internet for breakfast and your favorite series for dinner are therefore taboo. Even slow and enjoyable chewing is extremely important. The grandparents were right, as they had always reminded. Under no circumstances should you eat hectically between the door and hinge. The faster you go, the longer your brain needs to tell your stomach that you are full.

Grab your copy today!!!

www.ingramcontent.com/pod-product-compliance
Lightning Source LLC
Chambersburg PA
CBHW061712250726
48657CB00002B/604